Why Vegan...?

The Simple Truth

Robin Morris

Why Vegan…?

There is no copyright on this work. The author welcomes reproduction but due credit is required

Published in 2023

Robin Morris

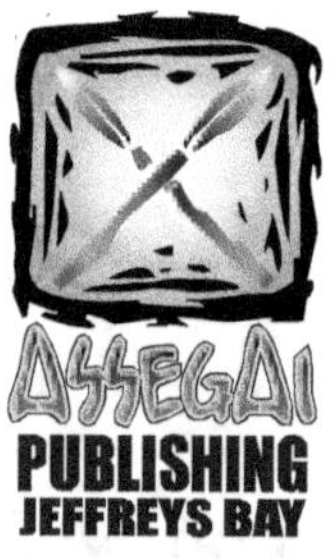

PUBLISHING
JEFFREYS BAY

P O Box 1588 Jeffreys Bay 6330 South Africa

www.assegaipublishing.com

*Assegai Publishing is based in Jeffreys Bay, South Africa. It is a non-profit organisation dedicated to spreading goodwill and spiritual direction via the printed word. All proceeds go to **J/Bay Pet Rescue** who feed and provide medication for destitute and abused animals*

Cover Design: Jimi Hendrix

ISBN: 9798371747365

I Rescued A Human Today...

His eyes met mine as he walked down the corridor, peering apprehensively into our kennels. I felt his need and instantly knew I had to help him. I wagged my tail but not too exuberantly, I didn't want him to be afraid.

As he stopped at my kennel, I blocked his view from a little accident I'd incurred at the back of my small cage. I didn't want him to know I hadn't been walked today. Sometimes the shelter keepers get too busy and I didn't want him to think poorly of them.

As he read my kennel card, I hoped he wouldn't feel too sad about my past because that's all behind me now. I only have the future to look forward to and I want to make a difference in someone's life. I know I can do it.

He got down on his knees and made little kissy sounds. In return, I moved my shoulder up against the cold steel bars to comfort him. Gentle, probing fingertips caressed my neck in return. He was desperate for unconditional companionship. A tear fell down his cheek so I raised my paw to assure him. I wanted him to know he could trust in me. Slowly my kennel door opened. His smile was so bright; I instantly leapt into his arms. I would promise to keep him safe and always be by his side. I would promise to do anything, just to feel his warmth and see that radiant smile and sparkle in his eyes.

He was so fortunate he came down my corridor today. There are so many more out there who haven't walked these corridors. There are so many more humans still to be saved.

Glad I was able to save one today...Fido

Contents

For Irma and her incredible team, who devote their time and energy to saving destitute animals in the surrounding townships of Jeffreys Bay...

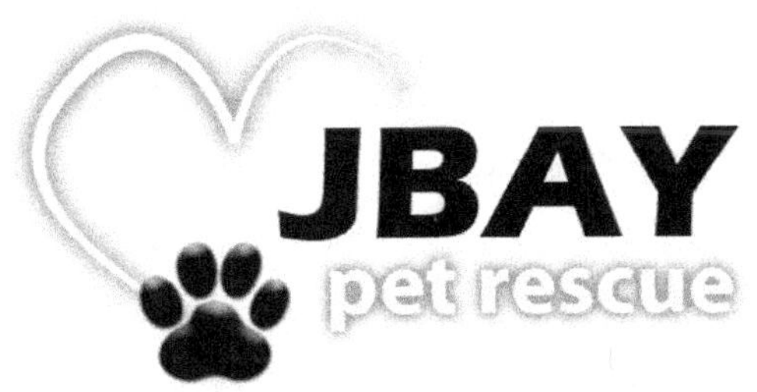

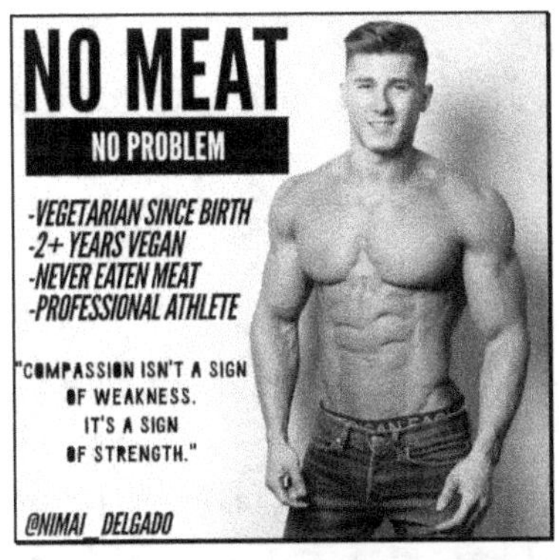

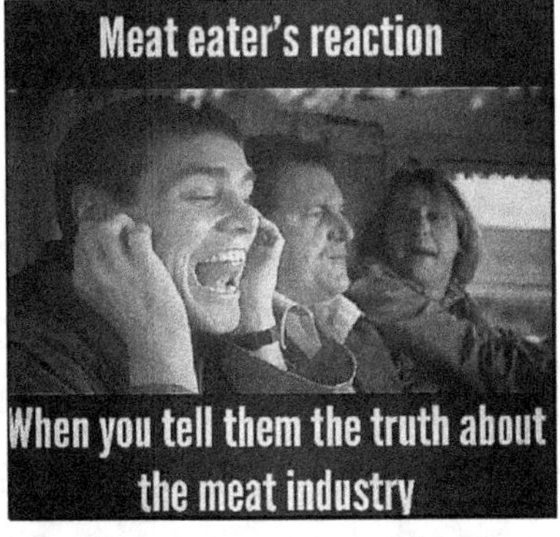

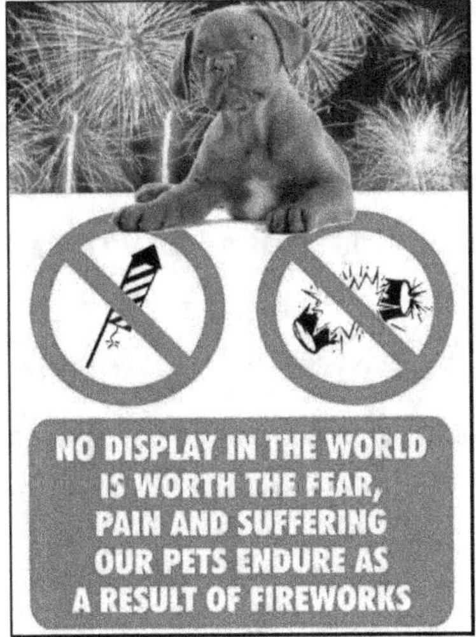

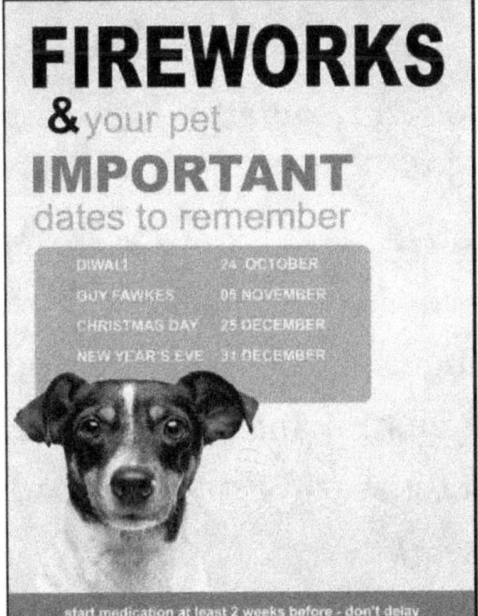

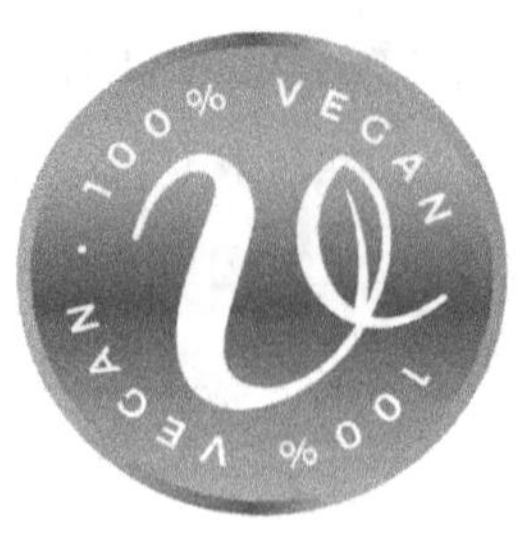

Balance...

'Veganism is not a sacrifice, it's a joy'
Gary L. Francione

Back in the day, Earl and Bart met for their usual once a month business update. 'So, Bart, what's currently going down that's new and exciting in the international business arena…? Things are kinda quiet here in New York. Hope you got something good to tell me. I'd like to invest and make a bunch of cash like that last one we did with your coffee bean.' Says Earl, stirring his fresh cup of coffee. 'Well,' replies Bart, 'this one's big Earl, in fact it's gonna be huge, worldwide. We gotta climb in now and tie up the rights for the USA market before anybody beats us to it because this one's already gaining ground in parts of Asia…!'

'What is it…?" Earl snaps, excitedly.

'Well Earl, there's this African animal, they call it a cow. It's a very meek and mild animal, has the most adorable eyes. Every time it has a baby, you take the baby away from the mother and drink all the mother's milk. When it can no longer have babies, you murder it and eat it. This one's gonna go all the way Earl.'

'Sounds revolting Bart. Must be side effects…?'

'Well Earl, because cow's milk wasn't designed for human consumption, when you drink the milk it clogs up your breathing system, your sinuses decay, it causes asthma, plus lotsa stomach and digestive problems from the milk curdling and rotting in your stomach.'

'Wow…! And what about from eating the flesh Bart…?'

'Aah, this one's not good either. Everyone eventually dies a wicked death from either a heart attack, a stroke or cancer.'

'You gotta be kidding me. How we gonna convince folk to do this Bart…?'

'It's all in the blood Earl. Once they've tasted the cow's blood, they're hooked; line and sinker, we got 'em. The big problem is, we'll need a massive and I mean massive amount of prime land for the cows to roam and feed, which means we'll have to wipe out all the Native American Indians and steal all their land.'

'No way Bart that's not good, there must be another way.'

'Well, there's another issue Earl; the cows fart and burp a lot, producing mountains of methane gas and cow poo.

The gas creates really bad carbon dioxide in mind blowing quantities, which destroys our atmosphere and eventually our planet. But no worries, we'll be long gone by then…!'

'And the poo Bart, what about all the smelly cow poo you mentioned…?'

'Aaahhh, as soon as it starts raining, all that poo mostly ends up polluting our rivers Earl. This is before it gets to the ocean and similarly pollutes the ocean.'

'That's sad Bart, so far I'm not convinced. Hope you got something else…?'

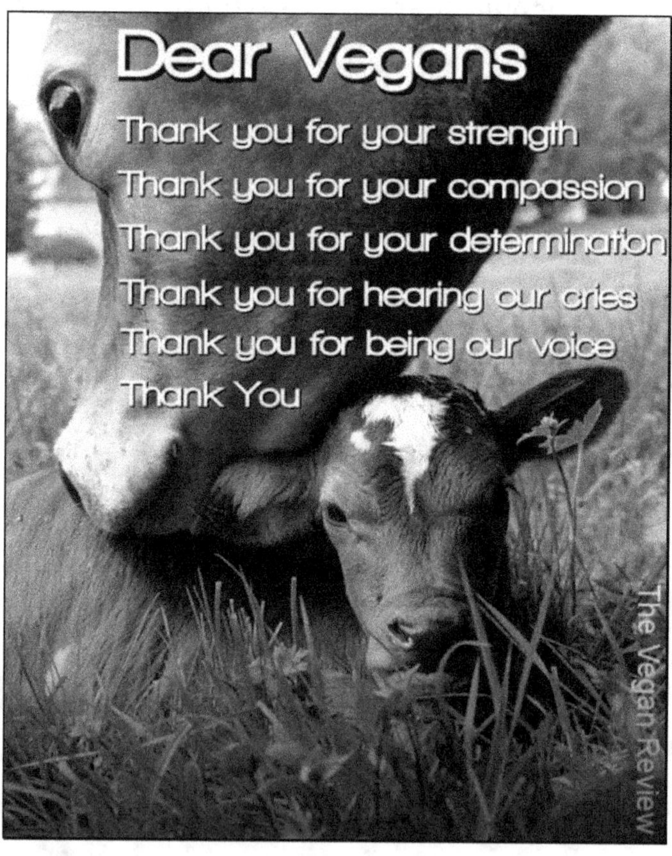

Okay, Bart and Earl, it's only a joke but a very deep, illuminating joke with haunting connotations and real-life revelations of man's terrible voracity over animals. Animals suffer every minute of every day due to man's insatiable greed for profit. And it's profit on a massive scale. We're not referring to the lone fisherman who stands on the shore and casts his line into the ocean with the hope of catching a fish to feed his family (although that also sucks…!). This is more about fishing countries who daily extract tonnage after tonnage of marine life from our oceans or large-scale farmers, farming huge ranches of cattle, sheep, pigs, chickens, turkeys and whatever else, for their skins, pelts, feathers, milk and most of all - their flesh and blood, for massive profits.

Sadly, the culprits are not conservation conscious either. They know full well the devastating effects they are having on our planet with their farming and harvesting of innocent life. They are no better than hunters or poachers (same thing really…!), who gladly murder innocent animals in cold blood with a high-powered rifle or worse, a bow and arrow. They somehow feel it's their given right to murder an innocent animal and feast on its flesh and blood, a flesh with little variance compared to their own human flesh. We are indeed, a destructive species…

Fortunately, there are those who have 'seen', realised all life is precious, all life has a right to live, all life begins and ends with God and therefore has an equal right to exist in

God's world and maintain life's balance.

Many guru's use the *'Three Roads'* metaphor to define balance in life. The high road is when life is supreme, business is rocking, your love life is solid, companions and fame are at an all-time high, etc. The low road is exactly the opposite; nothing works for you; everything is against you. The middle road is when you have balance.

However, one needs to initially experience both the low and the high roads in life in order to appreciate how special the middle road is. Mankind has travelled both roads for long enough to realise the middle road is where we need to be in order to maintain a reasonable balance in life and yet so many still choose the dark options.

The Chain...

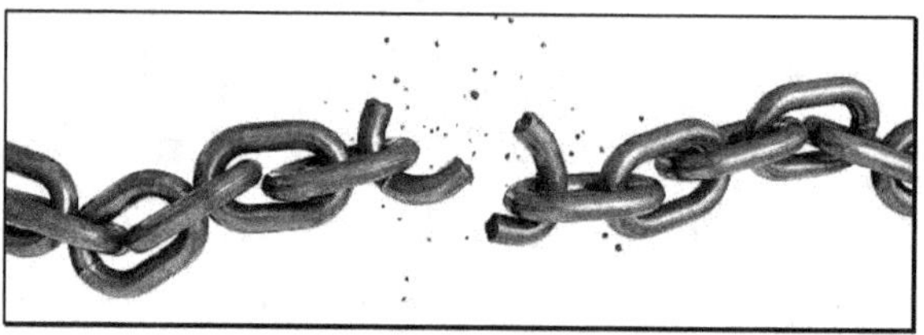

The story of the chain is a good example of how balance affects everything. A chain consists of several links making it strong and durable, each link depending on the correlating link it's attached to. However, break one link and the chain loses its strength and durability. The issue is, a single link has two sides with each side independently connected to another link. Therefore, losing one link, means both correlating links also become redundant, i.e. three links are wasted, not just one.

And so, it is in nature. Nature is perfectly balanced with an entire chain of herbivore and carnivore animals, marine life, insects, trees, plants, etc., all relying on each other for continued existence. When man interferes and exterminates links in the system, it causes irreparable balances to nature and our environment. Species become extinct, never to return. In time, all those species who were relying on the extinct species, now also tread the path of extinction and so it continues with link after link in the chain slowly disappearing. And all because man failed to live in harmony with nature.

Balance is all about Cause and Effect. Create mountains of garbage, murder untold quantities of innocent animals, destroy forests and their life-giving oxygen, etc., and there will always be an appropriate effect and relevant consequences. This is balance. We can't escape it. The obvious choice is to rather incur as small a footprint as possible on Mother Earth by living in harmony with nature. The simple solution to achieve this is to stop consuming animals, marine life and birds; leave nature to continue without interference. Harmony is bliss…!

'I see a world on the edge of a blade.
Without balance, it will fall' ~ Victoria Aveyard

Balance in nature is systematic, it flows naturally, like water, which is ever so powerful but ever so resourceful, it always finds a way to continue on its course. Take a bird, for example, it eats ants but when it dies the ants eat the bird. This is balance, this is nature, every species has a part to play, they know their boundaries. Unfortunately, man doesn't know any boundaries. Man, only knows what he can selfishly take and exploit for self-gain.

The Schumann Resonance...

As much as we have a powerful force of gravitational energy controlling the balance throughout our Solar System, likewise, it impacts directly on Mother Earth and nature with a magnetic energy force known as the Geomagnetic Field, causing all magnetic needles to point due North. This vitally important field is used by nature, humans, animals, insects, marine life, in fact, all life, to *'tune in'*, find balance and circumnavigate their way. Without this magnetic *'balancing'* effect, perfect earth and life as we know it, would no longer exist.

More than 3.5 billion years ago, embryonic life first arrived on earth. As primitive life evolved, it encompassed the earth's magnetic frequency and tuned in, essentially using the frequency to find a relative balance and for navigation. When human life finally arrived, another relationship began, a relationship that science is only recently beginning to understand and accept.

You naturally feel happier and more peaceful when you're out in nature, away from noise, traffic jams and neon lights. This is because when you're outside, breathing fresh air, with that pungent earthy smell beneath your feet or experiencing soft rain splashing on your face, your body tunes into the earth's frequency and restores, revitalises and heals itself. This is due to the earth behaving like a gigantic electric circuit. Its electro-magnetic field surrounds and infuses all life with a natural frequency pulsation of 7.83Hz.

This pulse (The Schumann Resonance), is named after physicist **Dr Winfried Otto Schumann**. The frequency circulates in the cavity bounded by earth's surface and the ionosphere, surrounding the earth. It plays an important role in atmospheric electricity and forms the inner edge of the magnetosphere. The area below the ionosphere is called the neutral atmosphere, or neutrosphere. Earth's electro-magnetic field is created by the clashing of the ionosphere, which is positively charged by the sun, and the earth's surface, which carries a negative charge.

Interestingly, the 7.83Hz Schumann resonance falls precisely in the middle, where human Alpha brainwaves and Theta brainwave ranges meet. This acute range of brainwaves facilitates a deep coupling of human physiology with the earth's resonance. These brainwave frequencies induce a state of balance, relaxation and meditation, enabling us to tap into the wealth of creativity lying just below our conscious awareness.

Pacific salmon are born with an inbuilt *'magnetic map'*

that helps them migrate over thousands of kilometres. USA researches believe the fish are capable of sensing the changes and intensity of the earth's magnetic field to establish their position in the ocean. They use the earth's magnetic field to create balance and navigate their way. The epic journey of the Pacific salmon is one of nature's greatest migrations. The fish hatch inland in rivers and streams, before swimming many kilometres to reach the open ocean. After several years of foraging at sea, they make their way back to the same freshwater sites where they spawn and die. Such is the magnetic influence of the earth's energy field...!

This same phenomenon, affects migrating birds and insects throughout the world. They cover vast distances, from continent to continent for seasonal changes, relying solely on the earth's magnetic field to attain direction and balance, tune in and reach their destinations safely.

Electro-Magnetic Fields...

Electro-magnetic fields are dynamic entities, causing charges and currents to move and respond accordingly because electro-magnetic fields embody and store patterns of information. They become a connecting bridge between matter and resonant patterns. The Schumann Resonance and the natural electro-magnetic patterns of earth, act like a tuning fork for all processes of life.

The bridge that connects resonances and brain frequencies, resides in our DNA helix, developed since early life began in the earth's environment. Ample anthropological evidence shows how humans have intuitively synchronised with the planetary resonance throughout human history, which is why maintaining a balance in life is so important.

Everything on this planet produces, emits and receives energy operating at specific frequencies. Our tissues, cells, organs, emotions and thought patterns, have their own unique electro-magnetic fields, as do allergens, viruses and bacteria. We tend to reduce our bodies' anatomy down to a simplified version, consisting of only flesh and blood. Grasping the intangible is something we cannot immediately experience via our simple senses.

It can be challenging to accept, we are merely a specific species (a life form – a sentient being), existing on this planet, just as every other species (all life forms – all sentient beings), equally exist on this God given planet. As humans, in reality, we are no better or no worse than any other species on earth. We were the last species to arrive on earth and may well be the first to exit, considering how we wantonly destroy other species, nature and each other for self gain and in the process, constantly erode our planet and the *balance* of its Geomagnetic Field.

Man-Made Electro-Magnetic Energy Fields...

It's well known, toxic substances (alcohol, tobacco, drugs, consuming animal flesh and dairy, plus radiation from cell phones, Gamma Rays from computers, TV's, etc.), distort the negative equilibrium existing in a living human cell. Due to these toxic invaders, the cell eventually becomes depolarized, losing its ability to magnetise and divide normally. The cells either die or they corrupt and divide abnormally, invading nearby tissues. These malignant cells then spread to other parts of the body through the blood and lymph systems. Sadly, these overwhelming cancerous cells multiply and kill their host, very effectively.

Bees (including many insects/birds/animals) are incredibly sensitive to man-made electro-magnetic energy fields. The **USDA** estimates, a whopping 80% of crop pollination is accomplished by bees. The busy bees are exceptionally important to Mother Nature in so many ways. Sadly, worldwide, bee colonies are currently collapsing, due to the effect of man-made electro-magnetic energy fields.

Physicist, **Dr J Kuhn** conducted experiments and discovered; mobile phone radiation as one of the major problems, considering there are now over four billion mobile phones in use worldwide. Man's interference with microwave ovens, X-Ray machines, mobile phones, especially cell phone towers, computers, television's, etc., have seriously clashed with the earth's natural electro-magnetic field, with devastating results.

In 2011, the **World Health Organisation** reclassified

mobile phones as carcinogenic to all life on earth - and yet we still use them...? Besides creating cancerous cells within, these man-made Gamma Rays also erode our immune and sensitive nervous system, to the point where a common cold soon becomes bronchitis and even worse, pneumonia.

Magnetism...

Magnetism in all its dynamics, embodies balance because it not only represents positive and negative forces of energy, it's actually one of the components driving our Universe. To understand this further, we need to look at how basic magnets work. A magnet has two ends, referred to as poles. One pole is called North, the other is South. Scientifically, these poles represent either a positive or a negative mode. To attract magnets towards each other, you have to place the opposite ends (North & South) of two magnets near each other. Placing like ends (North & North or South & South) of two magnets together, causes the opposite to occur; the magnets repel.

The dynamic we have here, is the *energy* existing between the two poles of each magnet. This simple yet powerful form of energy is infinite. As long as the magnets remain magnetised, the energy exists and it's perfectly balanced.

As an energy source, magnetism equally plays a significant role, even in simple everyday industrial use. A magnetised piece of iron (electro-magnetic) has the energy to lift many times its own weight. If you switch off the power and demagnetise the same piece of iron, it becomes just another piece of iron, unable to move anything.

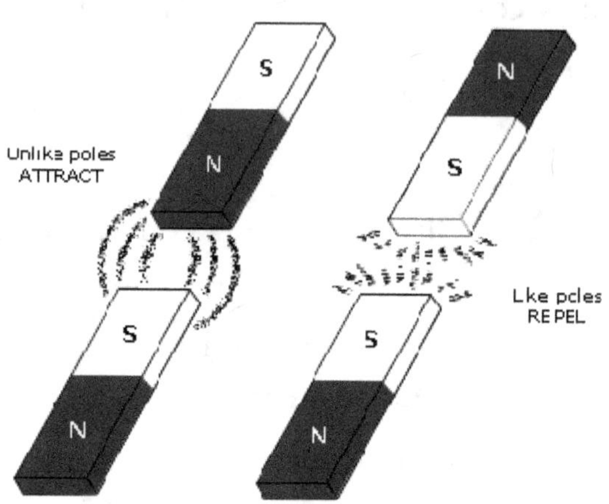

In Japan, they have high performance trains running on magnetism. Opposites will always attract. There's the story of the Swiss physician, Franz Anton Mesmer who in 1976 amazed the medical world, healing patients by stroking their bodies with magnets. Plus, we have the *'Bermuda Triangle'*, a region in the Western part of the North Atlantic Ocean (Bermuda, Florida and Puerto Rico) where aircraft and surface vessels occasionally disappear. Scientists believe this is due to an inordinate amount of magnetic activity in the area, affecting sensitive navigational instruments.

In a human or animal body, magnetism is the power source of the entire nervous system. Information delivered from the brain travels throughout the body in the form of electrical signals, called nerve impulses. When no impulse is transmitted, the ions outside a membrane of a nerve cell are positive whilst those impulses on the inside of the membrane are negatively charged. This positive/negative attraction then polarizes (magnetises), allowing the information (impulse) to magnetically pulse through the membrane and continue. Nerve impulses sent from the brain move at an astonishing speed of 274 km/h. Can't quite imagine how they measured it…!

This is *'Magnetic Energy'*. You cannot see it with the naked eye but if you drop a few iron filings between two magnets, you'll immediately see the push/pull combination. These mysterious effects also explain the enigmatic behaviour of molecules and how their atoms, consisting of electrons, protons and neutrons, create constant push/pull patterns of perfectly balanced magnetic energy within the atom.

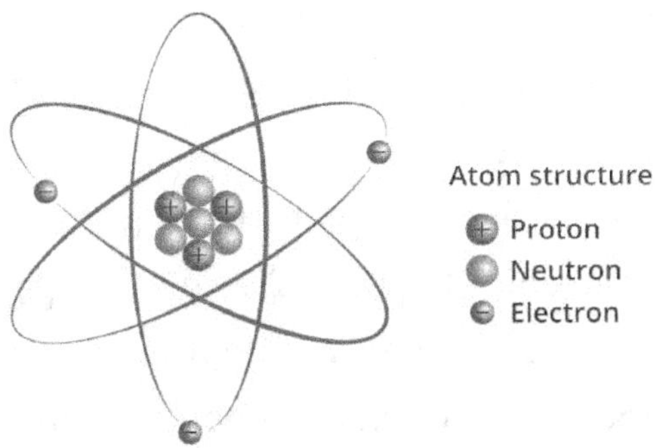

And this is the lightbulb moment - everything throughout our Universe, including all human and animal life, consists of atoms. Therefore, everything, is magnetically bound and connected. This is why balance affects everything. We're all connected with the earth's Geomagnetic field and because everything consists of atoms, (which consist of perfectly balanced magnetic energy), everything is automatically connected. Please, take a moment and mindfully absorb these phenomena.

A common example – when you're wearing a jersey and you unsuspectingly touch a car door handle made of steel and it mildly shocks you, this is *'static magnetic energy'* you are releasing. You cannot escape it…!

Yin & Yang...

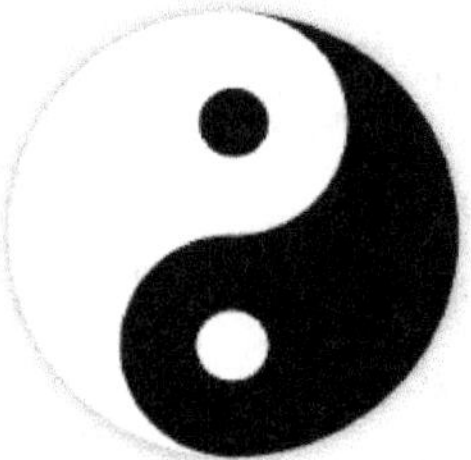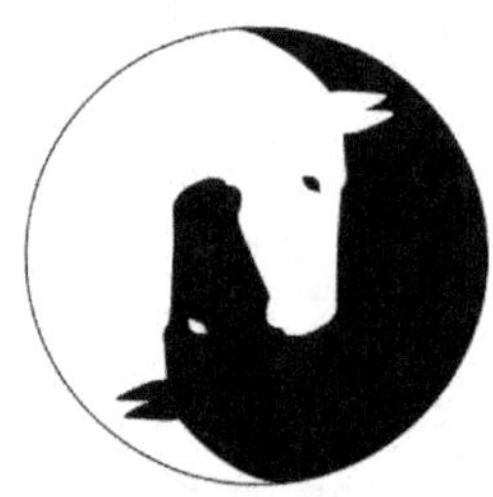

The Taoist concept of Yin &Yang is based upon the idea that two natural, complementary and contradictory forces exist in everything throughout our Universe, including all life. Yin is feminine and Yang is masculine or if you use our magnetic energy formulae, Yin is negative (passive and feminine) and Yang is positive (active and masculine). These opposite forces mutually complement one another, especially when in dynamic equilibrium. As one aspect declines, the other increases to an equal degree but is always striving for that harmonious equilibrium of *'perfect balance'* in the middle, which we all eternally seek.

The circle that represents the whole is divided into Yin

(black) and Yang (white), i.e., two halves in harmonious balance. The two smaller circles in the centres (the eyes), shaded in the opposite colour, illustrate that within Yin there is also Yang and vice versa. The curve dividing them indicates, this change is dynamic and continuous. Each half invades the other half, establishing itself in the centre of its opposite - *Simmone Kuo*

How does this personally affect us...? All life has their own unique, individual personality traits (their character) but they can also exhibit either Yin or Yang energies on demand. A person who is shy and inward has a Yin personality. An outgoing, assertive or aggressive individual is more Yang. Like animals, we all have our dark moments and equally, our vibrant good moments so our Yin/Yang personality changes accordingly. Most predator animals would be seen as Yang, whereas herbivore animals are more Yin but can turn Yang when necessary, i.e., under attack from predators.

Similar to the magnetic principle of North and South poles, if you place the same poles together, they repel but if you place opposite poles together, they attract. This principle of opposites and balance, equally applies to Yin and Yang, in fact it applies to the whole shebang because everything consists of magnetically bound atoms.

In life, a perfect couple (male and female) living in harmony, would be an ideal Yin and a Yang relationship, whereas having two Yang's or two Yin's living together, they would need to constantly strive for the middle point, providing some give and take, in order to find harmony and balance. It's no different in the animal kingdom. Coyotes; Seahorses; Wolves; Dik Dik Buck; Atlantic Puffins; Bald Eagles; Albatrosses; Beavers; Gibbons; Cranes; Barn Owls; Geese; Swans; Parakeets; Pigeons; Vultures; Angelfish; Condors; the list is long – are animals who all seek one partner for life. Studies have proven, a perfect Yin and Yang relationship exists with these animals, which is how they are able to stay together forever. Are we really that different from animals…?

This Yin & Yang balance of opposites likewise exists in music with song writing teams like Lennon (Yang) & McCartney (Yin); Simon (Yang) & Garfunkel (Yin); etc., it's everywhere you look. Even the relationship you share with an animal like your household pet, sometimes you connect on a deep level, (Yin & Yang) other times you don't, you're just buds (two Yins or two Yangs). Can't win em all…!

When the balance is right, all is good and harmonious, we go forward. Whereas, when one side of the scale is loaded, the reverse happens, we regress. And it happens in life and in everything we do. Whether it's the world, the environment or man's constant genocide of the animal kingdom, without balance, earth depolarises, progress is one sided, which means *one* has taken from the *other* and tilted the scales, leading to conflict, destruction, intolerance, disharmony, dissonance, etc. It's difficult to escape the *'opposite'* effects of balance...!

This is how opposites work. They create a balance, because almost everything ultimately revolves around a system of balance, or direct Cause and Effect, which is also another type of balance - the equivalent of ***Newton's third law: 'For every action there is an equal and opposite reaction'***. In the east, people refer to it as ***'Karma'***.

For human qualities, in simple terms, the balance is, whatever you put out you will receive in return, i.e. do good tidings with honest and open intentions and you'll receive good tidings in return. The more you wantonly give, the more you'll receive. However, commit to evil and harm to others, including animals and the environment and you will receive the same in return, usually with interest. And it applies to everything because it's all about the balance of opposites.

If we take time to pause for a moment, mindfully think about it and mentally come to terms with these phenomena, accepting there are magnetic energy forces of opposites constantly at play throughout the cosmos with resultant consequences for upsetting the balance, then we can use these vibrant energy forces to our advantage, merely by being conscious they exist and acting accordingly, realising full well, there is no need to prey on the sensitive animal kingdom in order for humankind to satisfy his/her fanatical craving for their blood. Neither is there a need to upset nature's balance purely for self-gain and greed because this will always incur consequences.

And So...

We already have Climate Change with Tsunami's, earthquakes, hurricanes, raging fires, extended droughts, a polluted ocean, ad infinitum, as man liberally upsets the balance, extending his destructive footprint throughout our planet, creating carnage wherever he goes, for maximum self-gain.

For continual survival, man needs to protect earth's existing magnetic energy field and not erode it with his manmade electromagnetic fields and especially, cease his abhorrent lust for blood and dominance over the many other fragile life species sharing our incredible planet, which he's currently exercising his right to selfishly do so.

Sadly, it's normally only at the end of our journey or circle of life, when we discover, all we seek is actually within us already. In reality, we need only awaken from our dream of separation and imperfection to realise, our spiritual God (the Universal Consciousness) is actually within us all. When you understand and accept this and that Oneness (everything is connected) exists, spiritual harmony flows in abundance. Sharing an elation of love and light, we simply co-exist in harmony with nature, the animal and marine kingdoms, with each other, with all life…the way it's meant to be…!

The following is a lovely story, which metaphorically explains this *'yin and yang'* concept of balance: At a certain college, there was a professor with a reputation for being tough on the scholars who believed in God. At the first class every term he'd ask if anyone was a believer and then proceed to degrade them and mock their faith. One semester, he put a question to the class:

'Who can answer, did God make everything…?'

A student raised his hand and replied, 'Yes sir, God did.' The professor responded, 'If God made everything, then God made evil.' The student didn't have a response and the professor was happy to have once again proved all faith is a myth. Then another student raised his hand and asked, 'May I ask you something, sir…?'

'Yes, you may.' The professor responded. The student stood up and said, 'Sir, is there such a thing as cold…?'

'Of course, there is. What kind of question is that, haven't you ever felt cold…?' The professor snapped back. The young student replied, 'Actually sir, cold doesn't exist. What we consider to be cold is really an absence of heat. Absolute zero is when there is absolutely no heat. Cold does not really exist. We only created the term to describe how we feel when there is no heat.' The student continued, 'Sir, is there such a thing as dark…?' Once again, the professor responded, 'Of course there is…!' To which the student replied, 'Actually sir, darkness doesn't exist either. Darkness is the absence of all light. Darkness is only a term man developed to describe what happens when there is no light present.' The professor was silent. Finally, the young student said, 'Sir, with regards to your earlier question about evil, do you really believe there is such a thing as evil...?' The professor smirked, responding confidently, 'Oh yes I do. We have rapes, murders and violence everywhere in this world. We are terrorised regularly with evil.' To which the student replied, 'Actually sir, evil doesn't exist either. Evil is simply the absence of God. Evil is a term man developed to describe the absence of a Godly presence. God did not create evil. It isn't like truth or love, which exist as virtues such as heat or light. Evil is simply a state where God is not present, like cold without heat or darkness without light.' The professor shook his head and abruptly changed the subject.

Nice story to depict the balancing concept of opposing energy forces. Without trying to confuse the issue, as already mentioned; as long as we have the *'one'*, we'll always have the *'other'*. This is how opposites work. When in sync, there is balance. When the balance is out of sync, there is chaos, which is why we need to find a consistent balance of harmony with ***'all life'*** on our beautiful planet, before it's too late.

The brain is the nerve centre of the inner self in animals and humans. This interesting topic is what we look at next...

The Brain...

*'If a cat does something brilliant, we call it instinct;
if we do the same thing, for the same reason, we call it
intelligence. How ignorant are we...?' – Will Cuppy*

The first time you see an anatomy of the human brain, its many folds and overlapping structures can seem very confusing, you may wonder what they all mean. But just like the anatomy of any other organ or organism, the anatomy of the brain becomes much clearer and more meaningful when observed in light of the evolutionary processes that created it.

According to *'Scientific American'*, ever since the first mammals appeared more than 200 million years ago, the cerebral cortex in the brain has assumed greater importance compared to the brain's other, older structures. Because these structures had proven their effectiveness for meeting certain fundamental needs, there was no reason for them to disappear. Instead, time (evolution) favoured a process of building expansions and additions to the brain, rather than rebuilding everything from the bottom up.

Scientists have also observed how the size of the neocortex has increased tremendously in primates, from the smallest monkeys, such as lemurs, to the great apes and human beings. Many scientists believe this growth in the primates' neocortex reflects the growing complexity of their social lives. Indeed, the ability to predict the behaviour of other individuals within a group seems to have attracted a large evolutionary advantage. Time obviously favoured the growth of the parts of the cortex responsible for social skills, i.e. language. These abilities were then improved as required. The increase in the folds of the cortex have also been a major factor in the evolution of the brain. These folds enable a larger cortical surface area to fit inside the cranial vault, allowing for a better organisation of complex behaviours.

Intelligence...

The cranial capacity of old Homo Neanderthalensis, the proverbial caveman, was between 150cm to 200cm larger than modern humans. Yet despite their huge brain, Neanderthals became extinct around 35,000 to 40,000 years ago, a time when the smaller, more intelligent,

Homo Sapiens shared the European environment with these giants. What's the point of having big brains if your small-brained cousins eventually outcompete you...?

Our ignorance, when it comes to how intelligence arises from the brain, is accentuated by several observations, i.e., an adult male's brain is heavier than a female's brain, indicating males are smarter than females. Also, in the neocortex, the part of the forebrain responsible for perception, memory, language and reasoning, there is a disparity translating to 23 billion neurons for men versus only 19 billion for women. However, no difference exists in the average IQ between the two genders, proving males are not necessarily smarter than females. Likewise, humans display more intelligence than animals but once again, it's a perception only, because it certainly doesn't relate to everything cognitive.

Our lack of understanding of the multiplicity of causes that contribute to intelligence becomes even more apparent when we look outside the human species. We observe how animals are capable of sophisticated behaviours, including sensory discrimination, meditation, learning, decision-making, planning and highly adaptive social behaviours. In labour circles, it is still common to hear animals discussed as if they were some inferior form of human beings, as if there were some kind of natural ladder on which human beings occupy the top rung. This is not what scientists see in nature. Every evolutionary species has naturally developed independently in order to meet their specific needs. Rats, for example, are perfectly adapted to their environment. They are not in the process of extinction; they live in perfect harmony with their surroundings and will continue to evolve and improve as their needs require.

Consider honeybees. They can recognise fellow bee faces, communicate the location and quality of food sources to their sisters via the waggle-dance and navigate complex mazes with the help of cues they store in short-term memory. A scent blown into a hive can trigger a return to the site where the bees previously encountered this odour, a type of associative memory that guides them back. This was made famous by *Marcel Proust* in his *'Remembrance of Things Past' (À la Recherche du Temps Perdu).* This busy insect does all of this with fewer than one million neurons, weighing around one thousandth of a gram, less than one millionth the size of the human brain. Are we really a million times smarter...?

The prevailing rule of thumb holds, the bigger the animal, the bigger its brain. After all, a bigger creature has more skin, which has to be innervated and has more muscles to control and therefore requires a larger brain to service its body. By this measure, humans have a relative brain-to-body mass of about 2 percent.

Smugness is not in store, though. We are outclassed by shrews, molelike mammals, whose brain takes up about ten percent of their entire body mass. Even some birds beat us on this measure. Humans still have so much to learn from nature.

People forever ask, what is it that distinguishes humans from all other animals, on the supposition that this one magical property would explain our evolutionary success, i.e. the reason we can build vast cities, put people on the moon and so on. For a while it was assumed the secret ingredient in the human brain could be a particular type of neuron but we now know, not only great apes but also whales, dolphins and elephants have these neurons in their frontal cortex. So, it is not brain size, relative brain size or the absolute number of neurons that distinguishes us. Perhaps our wiring has become more streamlined, our metabolism more efficient, our synapses more sophisticated. Question is - how did we achieve this...?

As **Charles Darwin** construed, it is very likely a combination of all these factors, including many more that jointly, over the gradual course of evolution, made us adaptively distinct from other species, i.e. walking upright, speech, communication, etc. We are indeed unique, but the important issue to recognise here is, so is every other life species, each in its own way, just as unique, just as necessary and vitally important to maintain the existence of life on earth. As already quantified, we are all sentient beings, all a divine part of the Universal Consciousness.

'Time is limited, don't waste it living someone else's life'

Frequencies

We have yet to fully define and understand the sensitive existential vibrational frequencies existing between animals and humans because animal vibrational frequencies are more acute and they obviously vary between species, some higher, some lower, depending on the specific animal.

Analysing vibrations is not that easy. It takes a well-developed intuitive sense to understand vibrational frequencies. We cannot see vibrations; we can only feel and sense them. People live by the old saying *'seeing is believing'*. It's actually the reverse. Believing will make you see. Most people only choose to look at what they know and what they can see. They rely on their five senses, unable to accept; everything vibrates, even our thoughts and feelings.

Think of a mother hen for example, with her baby chicks. As the mother scratches and digs around the yard in the sand and dirt for grubs, she emits a range of clucks and sounds, which her chicks immediately respond to. She uses a certain series of clucks for *'danger'* and a different series of clucks for *'I've found food'* and so on. Clearly, there is a definite communication/language /vibration structure in progress between the mother and her chicks (which proves consciousness exists in all animals). The clucks she emits are high or low, short or long, they're all different. Each series of clucks represents energy vibrations, expressed in wave formats. The vibration is the energy wave transporting the sound you hear. The frequency is the pitch. In this situation, you also have rhythm because of the pitch and then there is also sound, which now introduces modulation, which is about strength and tone. It gets complicated and these are just simple vibrations. It's the reading of them however, that takes a little understanding and this is something animals do naturally and yet we humans have yet to fully comprehend this. Animals are far more advanced in this area because they communicate telepathically.

Senses in the animal kingdom are also on another level, in fact, several levels, above humans. A mother seal can identify her pup from amongst thousands of identical looking pups just by scent. Think about that…! Did you know dolphins are so smart, within a few hours of captivity they can train people to stand on the edge of the pool and throw them fish...?

Okay, that's a joke but dolphins are warm blooded mammals. They enjoy a high level of intelligence and superior senses. A dolphin hunts fish using a sophisticated sonar system. Cats hunt at night because they can see in the dark while bats 'see' in the dark using an echo system. Animals, insects and birdlife have an onboard GPS. They're all able tune into the earth's Geomagnetic field in order to circumnavigate their way around the world. Dogs can hear our heartbeats and sync in with them. From this, they can tell how stressed or how calm we are from our heartbeat.

In Japan, they have goldfish who play underwater soccer with a ball. Netflix have a documentary called, *'The Hidden Lives of Pets'*. It's a fascinating insight into animal intelligence. Definitely worth a watch. These sentient beings enjoy advanced senses, way beyond a human's reach. And yet, we still think we are the superior species...?

We conclude this chapter with an entertaining story about a man and his dog. It goes something like this - A man and his dog were walking along a road. The man was enjoying the scenery, when it suddenly occurred to him, he was dead. He remembered dying and the dog walking beside him had been dead for years. He wondered where the road was leading them. After a while, they came to a high, white stone wall along one side of the road. It looked like fine marble. It was broken by a tall arch that glowed in the sunlight. When he stood before it, he saw a magnificent gate in the arch that looked like mother-of-pearl and the street leading to the gate, looked like pure gold. As he got closer, he saw a man at a desk to one side so he called out, 'Excuse me, where are we...?'

'This is Heaven, sir,' the man answered.

'Would you happen to have some water...?' the man asked.

'Of course, sir. Come right in and I'll have some ice water

brought right up'. The man replied, as the gate began to open.

'Can my friend,' the man gestured toward his dog, 'come in as well...?'

'I'm sorry, sir, we don't accept pets.'

The man thought for a moment and then turned back toward the road and continued along the way he had been going with his dog. After a long walk up another hill, he came to a dirt road leading through a farm gate that looked as if it had never been closed. There was no fence. As he approached the gate, he saw a man inside casually leaning against a tree, reading a book.

'Excuse me...!' He called out to the man. 'Do you have any water...?'

'Yeah, sure, there's a pump over there, come on in.'

Answered the man, pointing to the pump.

'How about my friend here...?' The traveller gestured to his dog.

'There should be a bowl by the pump.' Replied the casual man. They went through the gate. Sure enough, there was an old-fashioned hand pump with a bowl beside it. The traveller filled the water bowl for his dog and took a long drink himself. When they were full, they both walked back toward the man standing by the tree.

'What do you call this place...?' The traveller asked.

'This is Heaven.' He answered, smiling.

'Well, that's confusing,' the traveller supposed. 'The man

down the road said his place was Heaven.'

'Oh, you mean the place with the gold streets and pearly gates…?'

'Yes, that's the place.' Responded the traveller.

'Nope. That's hell.' Replied the man, sighing.

'Hell, are you sure…?' Questioned the traveller, somewhat surprised.

'Oh yes, absolutely, that is hell…!' The man answered, laughing.

'Doesn't it make you mad, they use your name like that…?' Probed the traveller.

'No, we're actually very happy they screen out the folks who would leave their best friends behind…!'

Sadly, we do have humans in this world who would gladly leave their loyal animal partners behind, even locked in a car on a hot day, in favour of the tasty world.

Animals and humans share similar emotions. In the following chapter, we have a look at this sensitive subject…

'If you think being vegan is difficult, imagine being a factory-farmed animal' - Davegan Raza

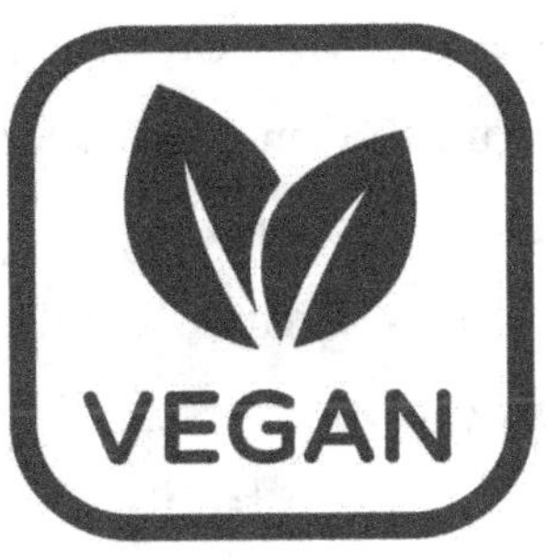

Emotions...

'Becoming vegan was the biggest change I ever made in my life and one of my greatest accomplishments'
Woody Harrelson

The *Cambridge Declaration of Consciousness* was signed by the world's top neuroscientists at a conference at the University of Cambridge, where world renowned, the late ***Dr Stephen Hawking***, was the guest of honour. The signed declaration declared all animals as thinking, feeling, creative individuals and consciously, human equals at soul level, i.e. animals are sentient beings with emotions similar to humans, able to express anger, fear, love, lust, happiness, humour, sadness and so on - they even sulk...!

As already mentioned, all animals are telepathic. Telepathic communication, or animal telepathy, doesn't require spoken words. For example: Horses are notably, intelligent animals, few among us will doubt this. As night descends, horses' group together in a field to sleep. They sleep standing up because with their large bodies it's more comfortable for them to do so plus they are then less vulnerable to predators. Remarkably, one horse in the group will always remain awake to keep watch while the others sleep. They take reciprocal turns for this *'watch'* duty. One can only imagine the telepathic discussions that ensue as to who takes first watch and for how long…!

If telepathy is the foundation in which all animals communicate with each other, then it is also how they communicate with humans. Animal Communication is a special telepathic ability we're all born with. This allows us to make a connection with our animal friends and enjoy an actual two-way conversation. As previously discussed, the ability to send and receive thoughts, images and feelings to one another is one of the oldest forms of communication. Many studies have proven, people frequently communicate telepathically with each other without realising it. It's how we make friends, keep aware of strangers and even fall in love. We're all born with this ability, this intuitive gift. It's simply a matter of relaxing the mind and *'tuning in'*. We subconsciously get to read the *'vibes'* when we resonate on the same frequency. And we can do this with animals.

Anyway, unless you have a personal pet at home it may be difficult to accept or understand, animals are an integral part of our environment with multiple shared emotions. Most people have at least had a relationship with a dog so let's continue to explore this relationship a bit deeper to provide you with a little more insight into animals and their sensitive emotions.

You can relate to this if you currently have a dog as your companion. It's an incredibly rewarding experience. Dogs have abundant love, which they share with you constantly. Their exuberance, deep emotions and love of life is intoxicating when you get to understand them. Dogs can pick up messages of scent carried aloft by the wind and are able to read another animal or human's Aura, in order to understand what the world around them has to say, making them very well connected with what's happening.

Dogs embrace the world and equally, the world embraces them in return. There are no hang ups, they merrily go with the flow from one day to the next. All they ask for is your love in return plus food and water and a roof over their heads. They want to be as close as they possibly can to you constantly, which many humans find irritating but when you mindfully realise the extent of their love, you'll appreciate and hopefully learn from it.

As a man, one of our pleasures in life is coming home from work, tired and weary after a long day, to be greeted by ecstatic children and yelping dogs, both of which are so happy to see you and share their day with you, all your work problems, which appeared huge at the time, suddenly melt away as you rejoice in the pleasure of your family. And the dogs are just as much a part of your family. You all share in the love. Dogs are not only man's best friend; they are protectors of the family. Most dogs will forfeit their lives without hesitation to protect any member of their family. This is because they are born with one of the most powerful emotions known, namely *'unconditional love'*.

It was **Josh Billings** who said, *'A dog is the only spirit on earth who loves you more than he loves himself...!'* Plus, they say the reason a dog has so many friends, is because he wags his tail instead of his tongue…!

Dogs have been blessed with incredibly acute senses. When they interpret you, they look straight into your eyes and read you from left to right, which means they first look at your left-brain hemisphere and then your right brain. They intuitively know, your left brain is your active mind and your right brain is your relaxed mind. By tapping into your Beta brainwaves with their acute senses they read you telepathically and it has been scientifically proven.

Obviously, similar to humans, some dogs are more

intelligent than others so the level of telepathic understanding between breeds and individual dogs varies. The average dog can understand a vocabulary of between twenty-five and a hundred words, depending on the training received. However, some highly intelligent dogs, chimps and even elephants, go above a few hundred words. There was one very famous and astonishing dog called *'Betsy'* in Germany, who developed a vocabulary in excess of four hundred words, which is quite extraordinary. If you think dogs can't count, try putting three biscuits in your pocket and only give him two…!

Even **Darwin** had a lot to say about the intelligence levels of dogs and their remarkably close association to humans. In the opening chapters of **'The Descent of Man'**, he brilliantly argues, using dogs as prime examples; *"Animals feel pleasure and pain, happiness and memory. They inherit a capacity for terror, suspicion, fear, deceit, timidity, bad and good temperament, rage and vengefulness. More significantly, they possess the powers of reason, imagination, love, jealousy and pride. They have deep emotions and even believe in the supernatural: There must be something special, which causes dogs to howl in the night, especially during moonlight, in that remarkable and melancholy manner called baying. Not possessed of human language, they nonetheless communicate. Who among us fail to recognise the meaning of our dog's barks, chortles, growls,* *bays, yodels and howls...? When in response to a whispered, 'Where is it...?' a dog charges from tree to tree, thus proving a notion there is something to hunt or fetch; this is indicative of engaging in abstract thought. Dogs and other animals, possess a sense of beauty or aesthetic appreciation, although mostly confined to sexual attraction. Their moral sensibility is manifest in their knowledge of right and wrong and their assistance to their family, pack or herd."*

Darwin admits animals may lack the ability to reflect on the meaning of life and death or their place in the cosmos. *"But,"* he then slyly asks, *"How can we feel sure, an old dog with an excellent memory and some power of imagination, as shown by his dreams and emotions, doesn't reflect on his past pleasures or pains in the chase...!"* **Darwin,** being a vegan, always expressed a sensitive feel for all animals.

Animals experience sensitive emotions, which are expressed instantly, unlike humans who sometimes bottle them up. Take a dog to the vet once and he goes placidly but take him back for a return visit and he will react negatively, even violently because he clearly remembers what happened to him the last time you took him; especially if you had his kahunies removed...!

These are emotions the animal's displaying. Unlike humans, who will first look for an alternative solution, animals react immediately. It's in their genes to do so, for in the wild, a split-second decision can mean the difference between life and death. Because of this, animals are blessed with super sensitive senses and deep emotions. Let's stay with the household pet for now and look at some of their emotions:

1. Love – dogs love unconditionally. It doesn't matter if you shouted at him earlier on for digging a hole in the garden, he still loves you unconditionally
2. Happiness – whenever you come home, your mutt is overjoyed to see you
3. Anger – mostly towards other dogs, cats, intruders...
4. Fear – the above visit to the vet is a prime example
5. Loyalty – your dog will defend you and your family with his life
6. Communicate – dogs bark and chortle, sounds which you soon get to understand, from fear to happiness
7. Competitive – if you have two dogs, they will be competitive with each other
8. Jealousy – likewise, with two dogs, there will be jealousy
9. Sulk – yes, dogs will even sulk if you've offended them unnecessarily. And so, it continues…

It's a similar scenario with all animals, not just dogs. Animals have feelings and emotions relative to humans. They may express their emotions differently but they still have them. Bear in mind, they don't verbalise in our language but their emotions can be just as volatile, especially with anger or fear.

And when it comes to senses (which create emotions), in all fairness, the entire animal kingdom equally boasts implausible senses and other extreme bodily capabilities that defy our imagination. Animals are on another level, way beyond a human's capacity and they use their senses almost on an existential level.

The majority of our thoughts consist of sensations, feelings, emotions, impressions, ideas and so on, basically random issues we think of in our everyday life, based on information provided by our senses. All incoming information is received via our senses and immediately delivered to the brain. Our senses are what feeds our consciousness. We need our senses in order to experience the outside world we live in. This process is the same for animals. However, it is the depth or sensitivity of our senses, compared to an animal's senses that create the difference. Let's take a look at a dog's six basic senses:

Smell...

Smell is a dog's most prominent sense. It is radically enhanced compared to a human. Science claim a dog's sense of smell is a hundred thousand times more powerful than a human. Dogs have around two billion olfactory receptors, whereas humans have approximately forty million. In the military, German Shepherds can pick up an enemy scent that is seven days old, if it hasn't rained.

Dogs also have an incredible memory. Wherever they go, they pick up various scents and remember them. When meeting a human or another animal for the first time, they will mentally record their scent. They will remember years later and identify this same human or animal via their scent, even though they haven't seen them in a long time.

A dog's keen sense of smell enables them to 'sense' some human illnesses. When we are sick, our body chemistry changes, causing the emission of certain aromas. Human noses may not detect these subtle changes but a dog's nose picks it up immediately. Capitalizing on this excellent sense of smell, dogs can be trained to detect specific **Volatile Organic Compounds** (VOC) in humans, reflecting an ongoing illness. VOC's are chemicals emitted by humans, existing in both gaseous and liquid states. By sensing VOC's, dogs can assist in the early detection of lung cancer by smelling a human's breath or even bladder cancer via smelling their urine. This incredible diagnosis connection between humans and canines may eventually lead to early warnings in all cancer patients as researchers work to isolate the protein or chemical, which mentally alerts the dog.

'A dog's keen sense of smell allows them to see'

Hearing...

Dogs have a keen sense of hearing. They are capable of hearing and identifying sounds over four times further away than the human ear can discern. Their audio bandwidth or spectrum, is far broader than a human's, allowing them to pick up extremely high or low sounds, for which a human would require specific high-tech sound equipment to hear and capture the same sounds. Their ears are also better designed to gather additional sound waves. They have fifteen different muscles that move their ears in all directions. Plus, they can move one ear at a time, independently of the other, to target incoming information. Animals who get agitated with thunder and lightning will begin fidgeting and shaking many hours before the approach of a storm. We can't hear the storm approaching but they have already heard the thunder from hundreds of miles away. Military dogs can hear the enemy whispering in their foreign language, in dense bush, long before their human handler gets anywhere near the enemy. They will also smell the enemy from faraway, if the wind is blowing in their direction. Animals respond to music. There are many 'YouTube' videos available online showing how animals react to various music genres. Dogs will often join in with a yodel or two…!

Touch...

Dogs vary widely in their reaction to touch. Some dogs

like a good, deep scratch, while others prefer a soft petting. Dogs usually prefer being loved and rubbed on the chest or behind the ears. Even a good friendly wrestle is sometimes in order. Some dogs get very possessive of their owners and will stand or sit on their owner's feet, lean against their bodies or walk in and around, through their legs. This gesture is merely showing everybody, this particular human is taken…!

Some dogs don't like to be touched on their paws due to sensitive nerve centres, allergies (grass and pollen) or nails, which have ingrown and need trimming. Please note – we're essentially talking about dogs here. Animals tend to react differently to various situations. A dog may prefer a good tummy rub from his human but doing the same to a lion in Africa will definitely have adverse consequences for the human…!

Sight…

Dogs have a wider angle of view than humans, but the field of vision from each eye doesn't overlap as much as a human, so less of what they see is in focus. This means they can see further around them. Dogs are very good at noticing movement. They're able to spot a rabbit twitching in shrubbery at a fair distance, which will be more of a blur to human sight. This is one of the reasons they respond well to training by hand signals. It was once thought, dogs were colour blind but studies have proved it's not true. Their night vision is typically better than ours as well. Dogs have an additional reflective layer in the eye that reflects light back into the receptor cells of the eye. This not only increases their night vision; it also gives the appearance of eyes glowing in the dark. Sight for animals in the wild, are probably their most important sense. Birds such as falcons, hawks, eagles, in fact, all predator birds enjoy a far more enhanced vision than any animal or human.

Combined with their other senses, cats have excellent night time vision. The differences in cat vision and human vision starts in the retina of the eye. The retina is the area of the eye where cells, called photoreceptors, are found. There are two types of these cells. Namely, rods and cones. The cones help to see in the day and detect shades of colours. The rods help with night vision and also peripheral vision (seeing from side to side). Cats have an abundance of rod receptors, but not as many cone receptors. This is why they can see well at night but are not great at detecting colours. Humans are the reverse. We're good at seeing colours but not too good at seeing things in the dark. The entire cat family can see in the dark. Lions and other cat predators prefer to hunt in the dark. Some insects can even detect ultraviolet light, which we cannot see. We're not quite as sharp as we think we are…!

Taste...

Like humans, taste is closely linked to the sense of smell.

This is one sense where humans excel over animals. Every dog, in fact all animals, enjoy different taste preferences. While humans have roughly 9,000 taste buds, dogs only have around 1,700 and cats only have approximately 470 taste buds. Every animal is different and they taste and smell their meals quite inversely compared to humans.

The sense of taste is a very exacting sense, sending a direct message to the brain. A human will initially rely on their sight before taking a bite and make a conscious decision because the signal to the brain is instantaneous. If it tastes good, they'll eat it, otherwise they may spit it out. Whereas, an animal, with their incredible sense of smell, will cautiously smell an object and decide whether to eat it or not. They either nudge it aside with their nose if negative or immediately consume it, if positive. They are seldom wrong.

'Nine out of ten people like chocolate
The tenth person always lies'

Intuitive Sense...

A sixth sense or intuitive sense, draws from the cumulative information gathered by the other five senses to increase the optimum level of awareness. Animals communicating telepathically with other animals, gives you an idea of how well developed an animal's intuitive sense is. Dogs, especially, have keen intuitive senses.

They read you like a book intuitively, immediately deciding whether you are friend or foe. It only takes an instant and he's read you.

Many pet owners have noted how their dogs are unusually intuitive. When we are happy, our dogs become equally exuberant. Ever come home excited after winning a tennis match or getting a job promotion and watch your dog jump around excitedly...? When we are sad, our dogs try to comfort us. Ever sit on the sofa in serious contemplation and have your pooch nestle down beside you...? Humans produce a group of *feel good* hormones such as oxytocin, serotonin, and dopamine. The levels of these hormones increase and decrease along with the elevation or depression of our moods. When we are sick, our dogs detect a fall in hormone levels and respond accordingly. As they comfort us, our hormone levels rise, we feel better. How rewarding for our dogs when they detect this rise in elation and realise, it's their presence that helped us feel better...!

Dogs quickly learn the routines of their families (or packs), the people they live with. They know when we are going to wake up, leave for work and return home. It's almost like dogs have an internal alarm clock. Ever have your dog meet you at the front door when you arrive home from work unexpectedly...? He totally knows your schedule. In one study, hidden cameras were placed in homes where researchers had owners come home at random times. Despite the change in schedule, the dogs somehow knew when to go to the door to greet them. Did their acute sense of hearing recognise the sound of their owner's vehicle or did they smell their owner's presence or did their sixth sense alert them…? Their senses are on another level indeed.

Our furry friends intuitively know what we need. But how…? Is it our facial expressions or our voice or our body language or our hormones or our smell…? It's actually a mix of all the above but mostly it's about the vibes. Animals are capable of reading your Aura and your reflective vibrations.

We may not be as sensitive as our dogs, but even mere mortals can recognise when a dog's sixth sense is activated. Service dogs respond, as trained, when their owner becomes ill. Dogs will also alert a person with epilepsy to an impending seizure or a person with diabetes to a drop in blood sugar and help them avoid injury by vocalising or nudging them to sit down or pull the car over to the side of the road. Dogs that detect changes in their owner's mood may cuddle up next to them or beg to be petted. Dogs that detect illness may lick the owners incessantly and stay closely by their side.

Mostly, you know your pet and likewise, he knows you. Pay attention to him, you may be surprised at how intuitive he is. Even though there is no scientific evidence regarding a dog's sixth sense, we certainly have sense enough to appreciate our dogs' abilities and how they integrate their other five senses on a heightened intuitive level, mostly way beyond our intuitive powers.

Some animals can detect forms of energy invisible to us, like magnetic and electrical fields. Others see light and hear sounds well outside the range of human perception. Scientists believe a light-detecting protein in the eye called cryptochrome, functions as a magnetic field sensor. Bees, can see UV light. Birds can sense when to mate months ahead of storm surges. Beyond echolocation, clicking and whistling, dolphins communicate with a variety of body language signals, including tail and flipper slapping on water, leaping out of the water, bumping each other and spy hopping. Elephants, communicate with low-frequency rumbles, called infra-sounds that travel more than a mile. Communication between elephants includes touching, visual displays, vocalisations, seismic vibrations and semiochemicals, which is a pheromone that conveys a signal from one organism to another so as to modify the behaviour of the recipient organism.

Dogs and especially cats, are able to see spirits from the *'Other Side'*. Think of it more like your cat is someone in your home, blessed with super powers. They can see and communicate with spirits we cannot see. There's the epic story of Rebecca (Quora), who was with her close friend when she died. Her two cats watched her spirit fly around the room for over forty minutes. She says, with both cat's heads, it was as if they were on a swivel, looking up, then down, then around as her friend's spirit flew around the room. Rebecca says she couldn't see the spirit but the two cats definitely did.

Animals have varied ways of expressing their emotions. Buck shed a tear from pain at the moment of death when shot by a selfless hunter. And then there's the fisherman who hooks a fish and after a long, gruelling fight, pulls it ashore. The fish always displays those large round eyes full of surprise (emotion). Sadly, the ignorant fisherman fails to see the look of bewilderment in those innocent eyes or the intense pain and suffering, the gasping for air or the urgent flapping of his tail (deep emotions). Somehow, the fisherman feels absolved of this slow, hideous death, committed via his now blood-stained hands. He fails to see the innocent life he has taken from this precious soul. It's almost like he's wearing blinkers and cannot see, cannot understand the emotions the fish is so vividly displaying right before his eyes.

Although animals have emotions similar to humans, animals don't carry the same amount of emotional *'baggage'* as humans. They don't gossip, betray you, plot someone's downfall or discuss you behind your back (what you see is what you get). There's no smoke screen in their world.

Temple Grandin *(PHD Dept. of Animal Science, Colorado University),* specialises in animal behaviour but sadly suffers from Autism. He thinks in pictures (Subconscious mind), which he says proves language is not necessary to form thoughts. Based on this concept, he conducted extensive research using various animals and birds in maze passage circuits and concluded that animals and birds also think in pictures. He could obviously relate to this. He further stated, warm-blooded animals definitely have a higher level of consciousness than cold-blooded reptiles. In addition, the level of intelligence in individual animals varies considerably. Carnivore animals when hunting, have the ability to anticipate their prey's next move, proving they are capable of thinking logically, like thinking ahead with the ability to weigh up various options. Likewise, herbivores trying to escape will use several alternative methods and make split second decisions, even resorting to the use of subtle decoys, which is quite remarkable.

Surely, by now you accept, animals have equally been created via the Universal Consciousness (God), but are merely a different species and yes, humans are more intelligent, because we have verbal communication. We can put man on the moon, build cities, etc., but then we also wantonly destroy Mother Earth and each other for greed and self-gain. This is something animals don't do. In addition, animals have these incredible attributes, like ultra-keen senses, where humans totally pale in comparison.

Fact is – we are all unique, we all belong to a specific species but we're all a part of the complete Universal Consciousness, none better or none worse. We all have a part to play. If mankind removes the animals from Mother Earth or upsets the balance in any way, the world as we know it, collapses. Think about that next time, before you consume an innocent animal's warm flesh and blood.

Human flesh, blood and bones are not that different to animal flesh, blood and bones either. Human DNA and Animal DNA are like every other living entity's DNA. It all consists of the same building blocks, i.e. A's, T's, G's, and C's. It's only the order of the building blocks that vary. In other words, a human's DNA has the same identical building blocks as any other living entity on earth but they are arranged in a different manner for each and every species. This is why you often hear of animals being grouped into specific families. It's because their DNA's have a similar alignment.

Ever since researchers sequenced the chimp genome in 2005, they have known, humans share about 99% of their DNA with chimpanzees, making them our closest living relatives. The remainder of the animal kingdom are not that far off. The genetic DNA similarity between pigs and human beings is 98%. Interspecies organ transplant activities between humans and pigs have even taken place, called *'Xenotransplants'*. Our feline friends share 90% of homologous genes with us, with dogs it's 82%, 80% with cows, 69% with rats and 67% with mice and so it goes on and on...

When it comes down to the blood, all mammals (humans, animals and birds) are warm blooded. However, the percentage of the cell types in human and animal blood varies. In other words, the order is once again different. In humans, the blood vascular system is closed, whereas some animals have an open blood vascular system. These variances are fairly minor. The main difference between human blood and animal blood is human blood comprises haemoglobin as its respiratory pigment, whereas animal blood sometimes consists of other types of respiratory pigments as well as haemoglobin. Sheep blood is the closest to human blood.

If you're that hooked on animal blood, i.e. cows, sheep, pigs, chickens (all mammals), then you may as well eat humans as well because the difference as you can see, is in fact, minimal. The next time you're feasting in a foreign restaurant, be aware because you have absolutely no idea what you're eating…!

Extremely gross to even consider eating humans but you need to understand, the biological differences between animals and humans are negligible, so why do we find eating humans gross but will willingly tuck into eating a warm blooded, sentient being, with emotions, feelings and senses, like a cow, a sheep, a pig or a bird and think it's okay...? Fact is – it's not okay.

At the end of the day, we're all a definitive part of the same creator. It's no wonder we all share a large percentage of the same DNA, blood groups, etc. We all breathe the same air, consume food and water to survive, urinate, defecate, copulate, proliferate, sleep and whatever else, to experience a God given life on Mother Earth. And yes, predator animals consume herbivore animals to create the balance but here's the truth – humans are actually herbivore and all we do is completely upset the balance.

Re humans being herbivores - consider the following: Animals and humans are mammals. Mammals are a warm-blooded species, consisting mostly of two variations, namely: Herbivores & Carnivores. The most powerful animals in the world are all herbivores i.e. elephant; buffalo; rhino; etc., so don't let anyone tell you, if you don't eat animals then you won't have any strength...!

Human bodies are designed like herbivores, not carnivores. Carnivores are equipped with razor sharp teeth and claws for killing prey and tearing large chunks of flesh off their victims. They swallow those big chunks whole, no chewing. They also have a short, fat intestine with extremely powerful stomach juices to break down the tough, raw flesh and digest it and they digest their food fairly quickly.

Herbivores don't have large, sharp teeth or claws. They have blunt teeth like humans. Humans have canine/incisor teeth but they could hardly be used for killing an animal. They are however excellent for biting into an apple, carrot or similar, which is what they were designed for. Herbivores *'chew the cud'* masticating their food into tiny digestible mouthfuls, just like humans. They have a long intestine with a complex and elongated digestive process, taking forty-eight hours and sometimes even longer to digest their food, just like humans. Obviously, our Creator designed the human form to be herbivore and not carnivore.

'Animals are such agreeable friends, they ask no questions; they pass no criticisms' - George Eliot

We conclude this *'emotional'* chapter with a fun story about a tired old dog…

An old tired-looking dog wanders into a guy's yard. He examines the dog's collar and feels his well-fed belly and knows the dog has a home. The dog follows him into the house, goes down the hall, jumps on the couch, gets comfortable and falls asleep. The man thinks it's rather odd, but lets him sleep. After about an hour the dog wakes up, walks to the door and the guy lets him out. The dog wags his tale and leaves. The next day the dog comes back and scratches at the door. The guy opens the door, the dog comes in, goes down the hall, jumps on the couch, gets comfortable and falls asleep again. The man lets him sleep. After about an hour the dog wakes up, walks to the door and the guy lets him out. The dog wags his tale and leaves. This goes on for days. The guy grows really curious, so he pins a note on the dog's collar: 'Your dog has been taking a nap at my house every day.' The next day the dog arrives with another note pinned to his collar: 'He lives in a home with four children, he's trying to catch up on his sleep. Can I come with him tomorrow…?'

Lovely light-hearted story depicting the independence of animals and how they always try and find a way to improve their well-being…

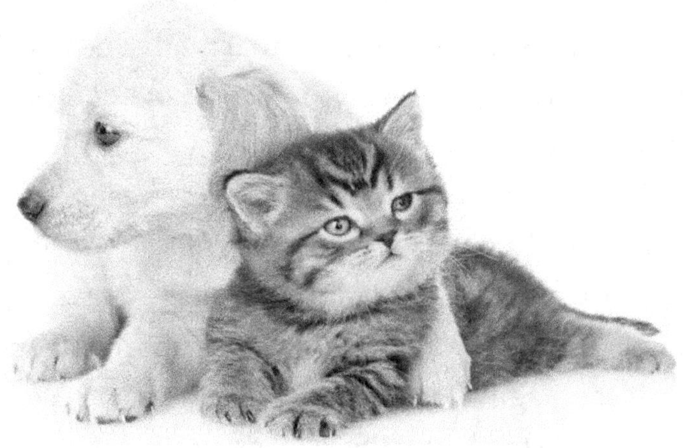

'Dogs do speak, but only to those who know how to listen'

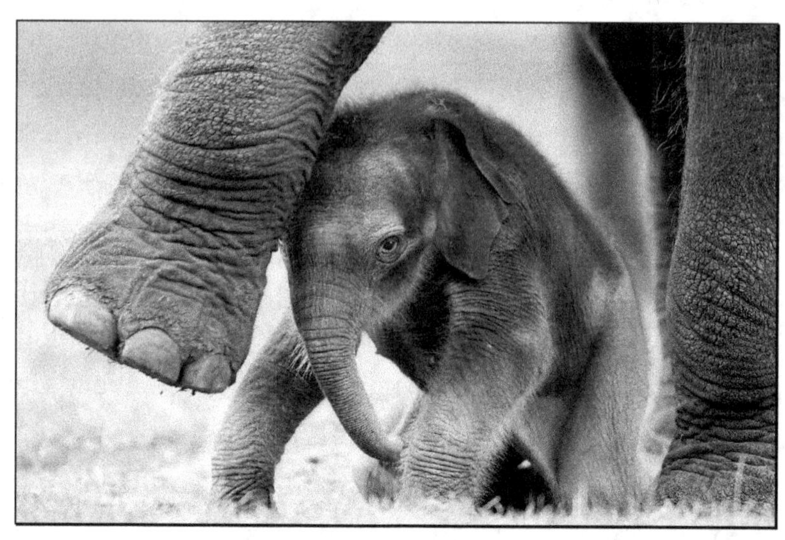

Animals

'All the animals ever eaten were once a mother's child'
- Buddha -

Biblically, God gave man dominion over all living things (*Book of Genesis*) but dominion actually means: *'To ensure the survival and well-being of all living things.'* In other words - Caretaker. No matter your religion, it still applies. Therefore, one of our responsibilities as Dominion Keeper or Caretaker is to ensure the co-existence between earth and nature is always maintained. This is one of the reasons why we shouldn't interfere or leave damaging footprints. We need to co-exist, not destroy. Fishing out the oceans, killing all the animals, cutting down the trees, poisoning the environment and so on, isn't what we're here for.

What does this mean…? Simply put, if any of the major components of nature are deleted, the system collapses. For example: The North Pacific Gyre in the Pacific Ocean is thought to be more than twice the size of the USA, known as the *'Great Garbage Patch'* to Marine specialists and sailors. This vast patch of once pristine ocean is where the world's plastic waste accumulates and is still accumulating. The plastic slowly breaks down into tiny pellets, which are then ingested by marine life who mistake the pellets for plankton. This releases deadly toxic pollutants into the worldwide food chain from commercial fishing. This is our shocking human footprint…!

Once we've removed all the trees, we'll have no oxygen. Remove all the animals and insects and we'll have no plants, flowers or trees. Increase the size of the hole in the ozone and we'll lose our atmosphere.

We have been given a perfect earth and a perfect nature to caretake. We therefore need to collectively ensure the survival of this symbiotic nature/earth or we'll no longer have anything. Earth can survive without us but cannot survive without nature. Earth and nature survived successfully for billions of years prior to mankind's arrival. It can do so again. Mankind therefore equally needs to co-operate in order to *'Caretake'* effectively. We need to fit into earth and nature's way of doing things, not the opposite. It's all about synergy.

Once we've learnt to tune into the energy around us, we'll understand this.

Whatever we cut down, hunt, kill or destroy has dire consequences, not only for us but for earth and nature. We have already learnt so much about nature. The time has now arrived to connect with nature, tune into nature's wonderful energy and restore the balance. There is an intelligence in nature that brings balance and harmony to the mind, heart and soul. Nature expresses a consciousness that is peaceful and balanced in a serene way, a joy that is omnipresent, touching everything.

Nature's cycle of life, death and rebirth is effortless, without fear or intimidation, just a natural flow and order of everything there is. Spending time in nature can be a spiritual rejuvenation. Commit to this, it's worth it.

At the best of times, humans are strange creatures. We are the only species who kill and destroy out of greed and who willingly express a blatant disregard for our fragile earth. Unlike Mother Nature, where the warp and weft of life is played out in a manner of the natural order of things. When will we learn….?

This is a story about a shoal of salmon who, mistaking themselves for beaver, vigorously set about damming up a river. They however, find this task extremely difficult, even daunting, considering they don't have beaver teeth or paws but they plough on relentlessly for a lifetime, day after day to complete their mission. One day an enlightened salmon arrives and explains to the shoal, there is no need to dam the river because by following the river's flow, it'll lead the entire shoal out to the open sea and total freedom; a majestic place of unimaginable abundance. All it requires is for the shoal to stop blocking the flow of the river with their misguided efforts and archaic beliefs.

The simple message – *Go with the Flow...!* It's not necessary to harm anything in order to survive. It's also not necessary to destroy nature and Mother Earth, which creates blockages to our natural flow in life. Pick up and move on to that open sea...!

Domestic animals make wonderful pets and companions. They enrich our lives if only we'll let them. Unfortunately there are still people who willingly take in animals as pets and abuse them, show them no love, keep them chained up, fail to feed them or give them water, don't allow them into the house and when they've had enough of them, have them put down or given away, or worse – they simply abandon them.

Animals are not our whole life, but they certainly make our lives whole. People who chain up animals or keep animals in zoos or a circus are committing innocent animals with deep emotions and memories, to jail for life. It's the same for people who insist on keeping birds in cages. Birds are a delicate warm-blooded species, blessed with wings by our Creator, enabling them to soar through the sky at random, only to have man cage them for 'cosmetic' reasons for the rest of their lives. Shame on mankind…!

Research has proven, a fully grown African Grey parrot has the equivalent intelligence of a human toddler. They can learn several hundred words and use the words to accurately identify various objects and will respond to puzzle-like questions. There is no such thing as 'bird-brained' in the world of birds. Predators like eagles, hawks, falcons and the wise old owl have equally shown remarkable intelligence levels. Ducks, geese, turkeys, chickens and especially bantams make fantastic pets. They will respond to their names when called, with love and devotion. It's all about the vibes man…!

'I personally chose to go vegan because I educated myself on factory farming and cruelty to animals and I suddenly realized that what was on my plate were living things, with feelings. I just couldn't disconnect myself from it any longer.' - Ellen DeGeneres

Science and research done on the true impacts of animal agriculture are constantly growing. There is so much factual evidence available, proving why humans shouldn't be eating their fellow mammal friends in the animal kingdom but man over time has unfortunately become very accustomed to getting his daily protein requirement from consuming animal flesh and more specifically, the blood. Blood is the hook that maintains man's insatiable desire for yet more blood and more flesh.

The sad thing is, he enjoys eating the blood of another. Fact is, he's completely addicted to it. Although he'll seldom admit it, deep down, he has guilt feelings about the life of the innocent animal he is consuming but his blood-lust craving helps him to mentally shrug it off. Plus, eating meat somehow appeals to his testosterone male image, especially when sitting around an open fire, cooking a dead animal and consuming it with friends over a few cold beers.

Maybe this goes back to our human genes, the caveman era. However, man quickly forgets, the human race has substantially evolved since then. Archaeologists have also proved; early man was more herbivore than carnivore because their primitive weapons were actually incapable of slaying a dinosaur. Early man ate whatever he could find. They were scavengers. The little flesh they did eat was mostly scavenged from dead carcasses.

Eating correctly is critical to ensuring a healthy lifestyle and longevity. Animal flesh is difficult for our sensitive digestive system to process. It's also plagued with parasites, hormone stimulants and antibiotics, plus animals carry large quantities of foreign and very active bacteria that are extremely harmful to our digestive system. Over a period of time these alien bodies erode our immune system to the point of no return. The domino effects of complications that arise throughout the rest of the body because of this are at times catastrophic.

In the western world the three biggest medical killers are: heart attacks; strokes; and cancer. Whenever someone is diagnosed with any of these, the prescribing doctor's instructions are – *'No alcohol, No tobacco and No red meat'*. First of all, this puts red meat right up there with tobacco and alcohol as the *'red line'* danger killers but seriously, if these are the main causes of these terrible diseases (including Gout), why then continue destroying yourself by consuming animal flesh, knowing full well the detrimental effects…?

In 2016, the *Harvard T.H. Chan School of Public Health* released a study, showing how a plant-based diet was able to reduce the risk of type 2 diabetes by a third. Switching out an animal-based diet for delicious plant-based alternatives, reduced the risk. A whole-food, plant-based diet is rich in beneficial dietary fibre, antioxidants, and micronutrients low in saturated fat. This is excellent for overall health outcomes, whether they're related to diabetes or not.

We all know the sayings:
One quarter of what you eat keeps you alive, the other three-quarters keeps your doctor alive…!

Some people think a plant-based whole food diet is extreme. How this for extreme – millions of people a year have their chests opened up, a vein taken from their leg and sewn onto their coronary artery. Now, how many people think a *'heart bypass'* operation is extreme…?

If you intentionally hurt, kill, destroy, abuse, perform acts of cruelty, etc., on any life form in the chain, especially those life forms higher up the chain, like humans and animals, you immediately disturb the balance, which invokes consequences, which will eventually impact on you ten-fold, because once again, this is how the *'Spiritual Balance'* of our Universe works, plus you will have indented on our Creator. We were all created by God's divine thought, which makes every living entity, a definitive part of God's divine energy. As previously mentioned, we're all connected so when hurting another, you're also hurting yourself.

'Just as each of us has one body with many members and these members do not all have the same function, so in Christ we who are many, form one body and each member belongs to all the others' - Romans 12:4-5

Animal Farming...

A plant-based diet versus an animal-based diet goes a lot further than the terribly cruel consequences of the innocent animal though because there's also a humungous environmental impact caused from animal agriculture. Our precious world is currently running out of water due to animal farming. We're also running out of land, even the Amazon forest is diminishing due to animal agriculture. Animal food production is now the world's leading cause of Climate Change. In the USA, 75% of all antibiotics produced are used for animal farming. What are we doing…?

Note: Animal farming is not just about cattle, it represents all farmed animals.

The Summary of Estimated Water Use in the United States in 2005, conducted by the ***United States Geological Service***, discloses; animal agriculture water consumption as high as 76 trillion gallons annually. However, a distinction must be made between water usage and consumption. Hydroelectric power is one of the largest users of water in the USA, but actually consumes very little water. The water is used to power turbines or for cooling and is always returned to the source immediately. Whereas agriculture is by far the largest consumer of water because it pulls water from the source and locks it up in products, unable to return the water to its original source.

Growing feed crops for livestock, consumes 56% of all water in the USA alone. Approximately 477 US gallons of water are required to produce 1lb. of eggs; almost 900 US gallons of water are needed for 1lb. of cheese. It takes 2,600 litres of water to produce just one hamburger meat patty. Think about that in your next meditation session…!

There are approximately seventy billion innocent farmed animals reared annually worldwide. And more than six million of them are murdered for food every hour (sick, sick, sick...!). Livestock now covers 45% of the earth's total land, making animal agriculture the leading cause of species extinction, ocean dead zones, water pollution and habitat destruction. Between two and five acres of land are used to raise just one cow.

'To get mud off your hands, use soap and water
To get blood off your hands, go vegan.' - John Sakars

Animal agriculture contributes to species extinction in many ways. In addition to the monumental habitat destruction caused by clearing forests to convert land to grow feed crops for animal grazing, predators and competition species are frequently targeted and hunted because they are seen as a perceived threat to livestock profits. The widespread use of pesticides, herbicides and chemical fertilizers used in the production of feed crops, often interferes with the reproductive systems of other animals, birds and insects. These deadly pollutants end up poisoning surrounding waterways, creating further additional major environmental destruction.

The overexploitation of wild species through commercial fishing, the horrific bushmeat trade, hunting, poaching as well as animal agriculture's impact on climate change, have all contributed to the global depletion of many species and resources and still continues to do so every day.

A third of our planet is desertified, with livestock as the leading driver. Every minute, seven million pounds of excrement are produced by animals raised for food, just in the USA alone. A farm with 2,500 dairy cows produces the same amount of waste as a city of 411,000 people. The important difference lies in the fact that human waste is treated before being discharged into the environment, whereas animal waste isn't treated or minimally treated by virtue of the storage methods used before disposal.

The *'Environmental Protection Agency'* quotes livestock and their by-products, account for at least 32,000 million tons of carbon dioxide (CO2) per year. This equates to 51% of all worldwide greenhouse gas emissions, which is more than the combined exhaust emissions from global transportation. The bad news is these gases stay in the atmosphere for a gob smacking 150 years. Even without fossil fuels, we will exceed our 565 gigatons CO2e limit by 2030 and all this from raising animals for human consumption. In addition, there's no sustainable way in the future, to raise sufficient animal feed to meet the world's growing animal flesh demand. Whereas, reducing methane emissions would create tangible benefits globally, almost immediately.

The *United Nations Food and Agriculture Organization* claims, we could see fishless oceans as early as 2048 with the current fishing rate of 2.7 trillion animals pulled from our oceans each year. Plus, for every one pound of fish caught, up to five pounds of unintended marine species are caught and sadly discarded as by-kill. Scientists estimate as many as 650,000 whales, dolphins, seals and sharks are killed every year by fishing vessels and that doesn't include countries like Japan, Norway, Iceland and the Faroe Islands who still in this day and age, hunt innocent whales, dolphins and sharks. Have no doubt, the Universal Spiritual Balance will ensure these countries pay dearly for their bloodlust crimes.

China is top of the animal abuse list for unashamedly plundering the world's oceans, as well as total destruction of many forests, throughout Africa, for Rosewood and other rare indigenous woods, including minerals and whatever else they can access. And then there is the exotic livestock trade, like even harmless Pangolins, smuggled into China and eaten. There is no life form safe from this nation. They will access, demolish and devour almost any life form in staggering quantities and they keep animals in the most appalling conditions. More in-depth info on these horrific circumstances in a later chapter…

Until one has loved an animal, a part of one's soul remains unawaken' - Anatole France

The good news is, we are currently growing enough plant-based food to feed ten billion people. The USA alone could feed 800 million people with the grain they currently feed to livestock. Meaning, if we stopped animal agriculture farming, we could easily feed everybody on our planet. Nobody would go to bed at night hungry.

Currently, as many as 82% of starving children live in countries where ample food is fed to animals. The fattened animals are then cruelly shipped to wealthy western countries for maximum profit where they are murdered and consumed.

We can produce fifteen times more protein on any given area of land with plants (soya, beans, nuts, legumes, whole grains) as opposed to cows. The protein content per acre of soybeans is 514,836g per acre whereas the protein content per acre of beef is only 19,544.7g per acre. Potatoes can produce 50,000lbs of heathy potatoes per acre.

Each day, a person who eats a plant-based diet saves 1,100 gallons of water, 45 pounds of grain, 30sq. feet of forested land, 20lbs of CO2 equivalent and one innocent animal's life. Take a minute and digest that…! Do you really want to be a part of this incredible destruction happening every day throughout our world…?

Farm animals are not future Buddhas donating their flesh out of compassion for those of us who have developed a blood lust craving for it. They are victims of our greed from whom we steal the most precious gift any of us has, i.e. *'Life'*. Animals of the world exist for their own reasons. God never created animals for humans any more than black people were made for whites or women for men.

With time, one becomes more conscious of foods that bring a consistent sense of well-being as opposed to those that make you feel miserable after you've eaten them. Be bold and get your health on line by cutting animals, fish, birds and dairy out of your diet. Not only will this physically benefit you, psychologically you'll feel like you've made a resounding commitment to yourself, Mother Nature and the environment. The first meal you eat, knowing no dead animals were used to satisfy your hunger, can be mentally overwhelming, giving you a huge spiritual high. Once you've taken this step, you'll never look back.

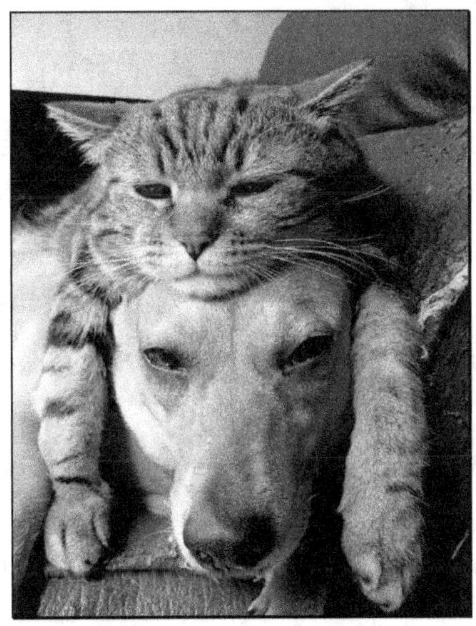

May all that have life be delivered from suffering' - Buddha

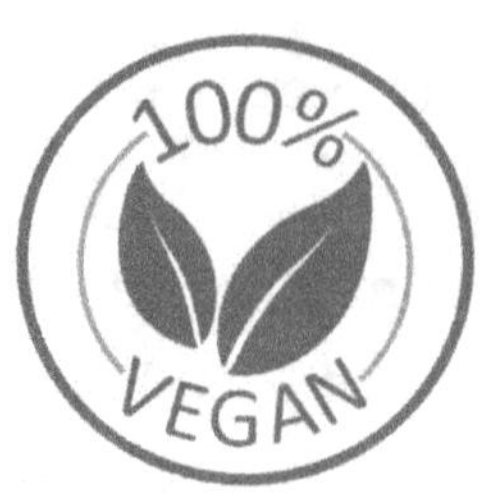

Religion

'Veganism is a philosophy, a way of living, which seeks to exclude, as far as possible and practicable, all forms of exploitation of and cruelty to animals, for food, clothing or any other purpose; and by extension, promote the development and use of animal-free alternatives for the benefit of animals, humans and all life' – *The Vegan Message*

This is a lovely story about Christianity and how Jesus gave his life to save his people. There was once a man named John Thomas, from a small New England town. One Easter Sunday morning he came to Church carrying a rusty, bent, old bird cage and set it by the pulpit. The congregation stared; eyebrows raised. As if in response, John began to speak. "I was walking through town yesterday when I saw a young boy coming toward me swinging this bird cage. In the bottom of the cage were three little wild birds, shivering with cold and fright. I stopped the lad and asked, 'What do you have there, son…?'

'Just some old birds,' came the reply.

'What are you going to do with them…?' I asked.

'Take 'em home and have some fun with 'em,' he answered. 'I'm gonna tease 'em and pull out their feathers to make 'em fight. I'm gonna have a real good time.'

'But you'll get tired of those birds sooner or later. What will you do then…?'

'Oh, I got some cats,' said the little boy, 'they like birds. I'll give 'em to them.'

John was silent for a moment. 'How much do you want for those birds, son…?'

'Huh…? Why…? You don't want them birds, mister. They're just plain old field birds. They don't sing, they ain't even pretty.'

'How much…?' John asked again.

The boy looked at John as if he were crazy, '$10.00…!'

John reached in his pocket and took out a ten-dollar bill. He placed it in the boy's hand. In a flash, the boy was gone. John picked up the cage and gently carried it to the end of the alley where there was a tree and a grassy spot. Setting the cage down, he opened the door. By softly tapping the bars, he set the birds free.

"Well, that explains this empty bird cage." John said to the stunned congregation, "but I'm not finished yet. One day Evil and Jesus were having a conversation. Evil had just come from the Garden of Eden. He was gloating and boasting. Jesus looked concerned but Evil eagerly rubbed his hands together and said, 'I just caught a bunch of people. Set me a trap, used bait I knew they couldn't resist. Got 'em all...!'

'What you going to do with them?' Jesus asked.

Evil replied, 'Oh, I'm gonna have fun...! I'm gonna teach em how to marry and divorce each other, how to hate and abuse one another, how to drink and smoke and curse, be cruel to innocent animals, feast on their blood and how to destroy the natural environment. Then I'm gonna teach these people how to invent guns and bombs so they can kill each other. I'm really gonna have fun...!'

'And what will you do when you are done with them...?' Jesus asked.

'Oh, I'll kill all those left over.' Evil answered proudly.

'How much do you want for them...?' Jesus enquired.

'Oh, you don't want these people. They ain't no good. If you take them, they'll just hate you. They'll spit on you, curse and rob you. If you give them work and wages to earn, they'll go on strike and burn your business down and then they'll blame you for everything. You definitely don't want these people...!'

'How much...?' Jesus asked again.

Evil sneered, 'Your life and when you die you must be crucified and die in pain and agony.' Jesus agreed and paid the price. John picked up the cage and slowly walked through the rows of silent people, out the door of the church.

Okay, we all love a good story, especially a story with all those hidden messages that make you think really hard about how you walk your path of light and love and how many innocent animals died today because of your lust for blood. When it comes to religion, another whole door opens because this has to be the most controversial subject discussed and debated worldwide. Let's begin with that wonderful end of year Christian celebration…

Christmas…

We all love Christmas time, the vibe, the coming together of family and loved ones and the exchanging of gifts on Christmas day, originated by the *'Three Wise Men'* who arrived bearing gifts for baby Jesus. What a beautiful concept Christmas is. Sadly, there is also a dark side to this wonderful occasion, practiced by Christians. Many pose the obvious question - does this concept really acknowledge the birth of the Christ or is it just a massive cash boost for the economies of the world and a virtual bloodbath for innocent animals…?

And how does a chubby little guy with a big white beard, dressed in a red suit, feature…? Is he the merry man who hands out gifts to all the children, especially the needy (we sincerely hope so), or does he merely represent the icing on the cake to boost further profits…? Apparently, he used to be dressed in a green suit until the popular American soda company, Coca Cola got hold of him and changed his green suit into a red suit, which was more in line with their brand colour…!

Is anyone even the least bit mindful, this is a time to celebrate the birth of Jesus or is it lost in the holidays, the financial profits and the Christmas dinner, where billions of innocent turkeys, fowls and domestic animals are murdered and consumed, creating immense animal hardship and additional wealth for sadistic profiteers…?

Truth be told, Christmas is a time for giving, not taking of harmless lives. The needless slaughter of animals and birds actually originated in the Jewish temple's way back in biblical times when animals and birds were slaughtered as a sacrifice, offered by the people to *'cleanse'* themselves of their sins. Obviously, the spilling of innocent blood in itself, is surely a satanical practice…?

'And Jesus called the priests and said, Behold, for paltry gain you have sold out the temple of the Lord. This house ordained for prayer is now a den of thieves. Can good and evil dwell together in the courts of God…? I tell you, no. And then he made a scourge of cords and drove the merchants out; he overturned their boards and threw their money on the floor. He opened up the cages of the captive birds and cut the cords that bound the lambs and set them all free' - *Chapter 72:7-10 The Aquarian Gospel*

This *'Cleansing of the Temple'* narrative tells of Jesus expelling the merchants and the moneychangers from the Temple. It occurs in all four canonical gospels of the

New Testament. According to the gospels, Jesus was horrified to learn animal sacrifices were still being made in the name of God, plus these innocent animals and doves were being sold by the moneychangers to the pilgrims because their animals had to be pure, with no flaws, otherwise they were deemed unacceptable, resulting in additional profits being made by the money changers who were charging excessive prices for their *'pure'* animals and profiteering unashamedly. Even the high priests during the first century seemed to have given up their love of God for the love of money. Apparently, due to *'tithing'*, the Temple high priests were wealthy beyond imagination. Similar to some worldly Christian Pastors today…!

Of particular interest, Jesus carried out what is euphemistically called the *'Cleansing of the Temple'* several hundred years after prophets like Isaiah, Jeremiah, Amos and Hosea had long since denounced the sacrificial slaughter of animals for any ceremonial or religious event. Christian scholars and religious leaders continued to ignore biblical denunciations of this bloody worship. They also tried to obscure the reason for Christ's assault on the system. They did this by focusing on the moneychangers, although they were only minor players in the drama that took place.

It was rather the cult of sacrifice that Jesus tried to dismantle than the system of monetary exchange and the blatant deception of the ignorant pilgrims. In all the gospel accounts of the event, those who provided animals for sacrifice for the Passover, are mentioned first. They were the primary focus of Christ's outrage. It is deeply disturbing to see Christian leaders joining hands across the centuries with their ancient counterparts to this day, in order to validate a system of worship in which the house of God becomes a giant slaughterhouse, awash in the blood of its innocent victims.

Animal sacrifices are a human way of transferring our own guilt and sins onto an innocent animal, which is then offered to God in the form of a pagan sacrifice. Not cool, considering God lovingly created every animal just as God lovingly created every human. We cannot scapegoat an animal to be a substitute for our own sins, for they are our sins and not anyone else's. The balance in life has direct consequences. Hail Mary's are not a substitute either.

"If only you had known the meaning of 'I desire mercy, not sacrifice,' you would not have condemned innocent animals" - *Mathew 12:7*

This is not about whether we should or should not celebrate Christmas and the sharing of gifts, it's about the needless sacrifice of innocent animals and birds at a time when we should be full of joy, celebrating the birth of gentle Jesus. For Christians, it is their given right to celebrate Christmas or any other religious festival for that matter; share gifts, spend quality family time together and praise the Lord but do so without harming anything or anybody, especially innocent animals.

Judging...

Our goal should ideally be to avoid judging anyone, even though the majority of humans have a difficult time with animal cruelty and the feasting of animal flesh, it's really all about personal choice. Understandably, once you've seen the light, it's difficult to comprehend how others fail to see it, which causes a deep internal conflict, knowing full well, everyone is aware of the terrible suffering endured by animals, considering they are also sentient beings with a soul. Your personal desire is always to set all animals free, safe from human cruelty. Unfortunately, this is a challenge we all have to face because we need to learn to respect (although it's very difficult to accept) the rights of others, who have yet to see.

Some people follow strict belief systems based upon their religious affiliation. Spiritually, this is perceived to be controlling and therefore unacceptable because forcing everyone to follow what may only be healthy to a small percentage of the flock, while the remainder go under nourished, is obviously not right or fair. Each to his own.

Personally, strive for a higher love in that all human life will one day get the bigger picture, set all animals free, return all animals currently held in captivity to their natural habitat and no longer consume them. The right way to change people's perceptions is to lead by example, people will eventually follow…

Animals, like all other sentient beings, deserve all the love and respect we can possibly afford them. We all need to live on this earth together in co-existence. We are not here to dominate any species. Rather, we are here to learn from all species, share and co-exist, in balance with nature. Sadly, we have not learned this. It's a simple lesson of kindness, decency and respect, for all life species on our incredible planet.

The religious practice of vegetarianism is strongly linked to a number of religious traditions worldwide. The following are a few of the more popular religions…

India

According to the *Food and Agricultural Organisation* (FAO), India has the lowest rate of meat consumption in the world. Researchers estimate there are more than 400 million people that identify as vegetarian. Plant-based eating is deeply rooted in three of the prominent religions practiced in India – Hinduism, Jainism and Buddhism. All these religions believe in the concept of *'Ahimsa'*, which means kindness and non-violence towards all living things.

Israel

Israelites enjoy a high percentage of vegans globally, with

around 5.2% of the population considering themselves vegan and 13% percent as vegetarian. Their increasing culture of veganism and the abundance of plant-based options makes it one of the best countries to visit for vegans and vegetarians. You'll find plant-based foods such as hummus and falafels at every turn and it's not uncommon for worldwide brands such as *'Dominos'* and *'Ben and Jerry's'* to offer multiple vegan-friendly options in Israel.

Jamaican Ital food

Ital, is the food celebrated by those in the Rastafari movement developed in Jamaica during the 1930s, based on natural living. Rastas are earth-preservers and believe the food they eat should come from the land. This, in principle, is Ital. Ital food should be natural, organic, unprocessed and free of additives, chemicals and meat. The name derives from the word *'vital'*. Combined with a climate well-suited to growing a variety of fruit and vegetables, this means there are plenty of plant-based options available in Jamaica and the rest of the Caribbean. The choice to eat Ital is as much of a spiritual decision for Rastas as it is a health conscious one. Their philosophy is to remain as close to nature as possible and respect all forms of animal and plant life. They believe eating pure, organic food increases one's connection with nature.

'No Woman No Cry' — Bob Marley

Ethiopian and Eritrean Cuisine

The cuisine of Eritrea and Ethiopia is full of naturally plant-based dishes. This is largely due to the fasting tradition in the Orthodox Christian religion. Orthodox Christians abstain from all animal products for around 200 days each year, but plant-based foods are still permitted. Many fast every Wednesday and Friday, during Lent, in the days leading up to Christmas and during other religious holidays. The tradition of fasting has been around for centuries. It's not uncommon for Orthodox-owned businesses, such as butcher shops, to close on fasting days; for cafes to not stock milk and for restaurants to offer a plant-based menu only.

Jainism

The food choices of Jains are based on the value of *'Ahimsa'* (non-violence). This causes the Jains to prefer food that inflict the least amount of violence. Vegetarianism is considered mandatory for everyone. Jains are either lacto-vegetarians or vegans. No use or consumption of products obtained from dead animals is allowed. Moreover, Jains try to avoid unnecessary injury to plants and subtle life forms. The goal is to cause as little violence to living things as possible, hence they avoid eating roots, tubers such as potatoes, garlic and anything that involves uprooting (and thus eventually killing) a plant to obtain food. Every act by which a person directly or indirectly supports killing or injury is seen as violence, which creates harmful Karma. The aim of *'Ahimsa'* is to prevent the accumulation of such Karma. Jains consider nonviolence to be the most essential religious duty for everyone, a statement which is often inscribed on Jain temples. Their scrupulous and thorough way of applying nonviolence to everyday activities, especially to food, shapes their entire lives. It is the most significant hallmark of Jain identity. Jains do not practice animal sacrifice as they consider all sentient beings to be equal.

Hinduism

Hinduism has a wide variety of practices and beliefs that have changed over time. An estimated 33% of all Hindus are vegetarians. The principle of nonviolence applied to animals is connected with the intention to avoid negative Karmic influences which result from violence. The suffering of all beings is believed to arise from craving and desire, conditioned by the Karmic effects of both animal and human action. The violence of slaughtering animals for food and its source in craving, reveal flesh eating as one mode in which humans enslave themselves to suffering. Hinduism holds that such influences affect the person who permits the slaughter of an animal, the person who kills it, the person who cuts it up, the person who buys or sells the meat, the person who cooks it, the person who serves it up and finally, the person who eats it. They must all be considered the slayers of the animal. The question of religious duties towards the animals and of negative Karma incurred from violence against them is discussed in detail in Hindu scriptures and religious law books.

Hindu scriptures belong to the Vedic period which lasted till about 500 BCE, according to the chronological division by modern historians. In the historical Vedic religion, the predecessor of Hinduism, meat eating was not banned in principle, but was restricted by specific rules. However, several highly authoritative scriptures bar violence against domestic animals.

Hindus point to the Mahabharata's maxim that *'Nonviolence is the highest duty and the highest teaching'* clearly advocating a vegetarian diet. It also states that sin was born when creatures started to devour one another from want of food. These texts strongly condemn the slaughter of animals and meat eating. In modern India, the food habits of Hindus vary according to their community or caste and according to regional traditions. Hindu vegetarians usually eschew eggs but some consume dairy products, so they are lacto-vegetarians.

Buddhism

The first Buddhist monks and nuns were forbidden from growing, storing or cooking their own food. They relied entirely on the generosity of *'alms'* to feed themselves. They were not allowed to accept money to buy their own food or make special dietary requests. They had to accept whatever food the *'alms givers'* had available.

Devadatta urged the Buddha to make complete abstinence from meat compulsory. The Buddha answered, 'How can the monks refuse what has been given to them in charity…?', maintaining, monks would have to accept whatever they found in their begging bowls.

Some Mahayana sutras strongly denounce the eating of meat. An entire chapter is devoted to the Buddha's response, wherein he lists a litany of spiritual, physical, mental and emotional reasons why meat eating should be avoided. In several other Mahayana scriptures, the Buddha is seen clearly to indicate that meat-eating is undesirable and Karmically unwholesome.

Some suggest, the rise of monasteries in Mahayana tradition are the contributing factor in the emphasis on vegetarianism. When monks from the Indian geographical sphere of influence migrated to China from the year 65 CE on, they met followers who provided them with money instead of food. From those days onwards, Chinese monastics and others who came to inhabit northern countries, cultivated their own vegetable plots and bought food in the market. In China, Korea, Vietnam, Taiwan and their respective diaspora communities, monks and nuns are expected to abstain from meat, eggs and dairy, in addition to the fetid vegetables – traditionally Garlic, Allium Chinense, Asafoetida, Shallot and Allium Victorialis (victory onion or mountain leek), although in modern times this rule is often interpreted to include other vegetables of the onion genus, as well as coriander. This is called pure vegetarianism or veganism.

In the modern Buddhist world, attitudes toward vegetarianism vary by location. In China and Vietnam, monks typically eat no meat, with other restrictions as well. In Japan or Korea, only some schools do not eat meat. All Buddhists, including monks, are allowed to practice vegetarianism if they wish to do so.

Abrahamic Religions

Judaic, Christian and Muslim traditions all have strong connections to the Biblical ideal of the Garden of Eden, which includes references to a herbivore diet - *Genesis 1:29–31, Isaiah 11:6–9.*

While vegetarianism has not traditionally been viewed as mainstream in these traditions, some Jews, Christians and Muslims practice and advocate vegetarianism. Some Jewish vegetarians have pointed out that Adam and Eve were not allowed to eat meat. *Genesis 1:29* states: And God said, *'Behold, I have given you every herb yielding seed which is upon the face of all the earth and every tree that has seed-yielding fruit, to you it shall be for food.'* indicating that God's original plan was for mankind to be vegan. According to some opinions, the whole world will again be vegetarian in the Messianic era. Not eating meat brings the world closer to that ideal. As the ideal images of the Torah are vegetarian, one may see the laws of kashrut as actually designed to wean Jews away from meat eating and to move them toward the vegetarian ideal.

Christianity

Within Eastern Christianity, vegetarianism is practiced as part of fasting during the Great Lent. Vegan fasting is particularly common in Eastern Orthodoxy and Oriental Orthodox Churches, such as the Coptic Orthodox Church of Alexandria. Some Christian groups, such as Seventh-day Adventists, the Christian Vegetarian Association and Christian anarchists, take a literal interpretation of the Biblical prophecies of universal vegetarianism (or veganism) *Genesis 1:29–1:31, Isaiah 11:6–11:9, Isaiah 65:25* and encourage these practices as preferred lifestyles or as a tool to reject the commodity status of animals and the use of animal products for any purpose, although some of them say it is not required.

The Bible Christian Church, a Christian vegetarian sect founded by Reverend William Cowherd in 1809, were one of the philosophical forerunners of the Vegetarian Society. Cowherd encouraged members to abstain from eating meat as a form of temperance. Some Christian vegetarians, such as Keith Akers, argue that Jesus himself was a vegetarian. Akers argues that Jesus was influenced by the Essenes, an ascetic Jewish sect. There is no historical record of Jesus' precise attitudes to animals, but there is a strand in his ethical teaching about the primacy of mercy to the weak, the powerless and the oppressed, which Walters and Portmess argue can also refer to captive animals.

Other, more recent Christians movements, such as Sarx and CreatureKind, argue that many practices which occur in the contemporary industrialized farming system, such as the mass culling of day-old male-chicks in the egg industry, are incompatible with the life of peace and love to which Jesus called his followers.

Islam

Islam explicitly prohibits eating of some kinds of meat, especially pork. However, one of the most important Islamic celebrations, Eid al-Adha, involves animal sacrifices. Muslims who can afford to do so sacrifice domestic animals (usually sheep but also camels, cows and goats). According to the Quran, a large portion of the meat has to be given towards the poor and hungry and every effort is made to see no impoverished Muslim is left without sacrificial meat during the days of feasts like Eid-ul-Adha.

Certain Islamic orders are mainly vegetarian; many Sufis maintain a vegetarian diet. Some Muslims in Indonesia think being a vegetarian for reasons other than health, is un-Islamic and a form of emulation of the infidels. On the other hand, the Rishi order in Kashmir were historically described as abstaining from meat consumption.

The prophet Muhammad, however, was opposed to the frequent consumption of meat and for his part, was said to subsist mainly on a diet of dates and barley. The former Indian president Dr A. P. J. Abdul Kalam was also famously a vegetarian. In January 1996, The International Vegetarian Union announced the formation of the Muslim Vegetarian/Vegan Society. There is also a Vegan Muslim Initiative, founded in 2017. They encourage Muslims to try a vegan diet during Ramadan, making it a *'Veganadan'*.

Proponents of vegetarianism in Islam have pointed to the teachings in the Quran and the Hadith, which instruct kindness and compassion towards animals: -

1. Whoever is kind to the creatures of God is kind to himself – *Hadith: Bukhari*

2. A good deed done to an animal is as meritorious as a good deed done to a human being, while an act of cruelty to an animal is as bad as an act of cruelty to a human being – *Hadith: Mishkat al-Masabih; Book 6; Chapter 7, 8:178*

3. Sons of wisdom, do not turn your stomachs into graveyards for animals – *Hadith: Fayd al-Qadīr Sharh al-Jami' as-Saghīr 2/52*

4. Beware of meat, for meat can be as addictive as wine – *Hadith: al-Muwaṭṭa' 1742*

The Nation of Islam promotes vegetarianism deeming it -
'The Most healthful and virtuous way to eat'

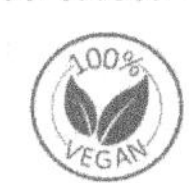

Bahá'í Faith

While there are no dietary restrictions in the Baha'i faith, 'Abdu'l-Bahá, the son of the founder of the religion, noted that a vegetarian diet consisting of fruits and grains was desirable, except for people with a weak constitution or those who are sick. He stated, there are no requirements that Bahá'ís become vegetarian, but that a future society would gradually become vegetarian. 'Abdu'l-Bahá also stated that killing animals was somewhat contrary to compassion. While Shoghi Effendi, the head of the Bahá'í Faith in the first half of the 20th century, stated that a purely vegetarian diet would be preferable since it avoided killing animals. Both he and the Universal House of Justice (the governing body of the Bahá'ís) have stated, these teachings do not constitute a Bahá'í practice, Bahá'ís can choose to eat whatever they wish, but to be respectful of others' beliefs.

Taoism

In Chinese societies, *'simple eating'* refers to a particular restricted diet associated with Taoist monks, sometimes practiced by members of the general population during Taoist festivals and fasting days. It is similar to Chinese Buddhist vegetarianism. Varying levels of abstinence among Taoists and Taoist-influenced people include veganism, veganism without root vegetables, lacto-ovo vegetarianism and pescetarianism. Taoist vegetarians also tend to abstain from alcohol and pungent vegetables such as garlic and onions during Lenten days. Non-vegetarian Taoists sometimes abstain from beef and water buffalo meat for many cultural reasons. Vegetarianism in the Taoist tradition is similar to that of Lent in the Christian tradition.

While highly religious people such as monks may be vegetarian, vegan or pescatarian on a permanent basis, lay practitioners often eat vegetarian on the 1st (new moon), 8th, 14th, 18th, 23rd, 24th, 28th, 29th and 30th days of the lunar calendar. In accordance with their Buddhist peers (because many people are both Taoist and Buddhist), they often also eat Lenten on the 15th day (full moon).

Taoist vegetarianism is similar to Chinese Buddhist vegetarianism, however, its roots reach to pre-Buddhist times. Believers historically abstained from animal products and alcohol before practicing Confucian, Taoist and Chinese folk religion rites. It is referred to by the English word *'vegetarian'*; however, though it rejects meat, eggs and milk, this diet may include oysters and oyster products or otherwise be pescatarian for some believers. Many lay Taoists who follow modern sects such as that of Yi Guan Dao or Master Ching Hai are vegan or strictly vegetarian.

Faithist/Oahspe

Oahspe (meaning Sky, Earth and Spirit) is the doctrinal

book of those who follow Faithism. The precepts for behaviour can be found throughout the book which include a herbivorous diet (vegan, vegetable food only), peaceful living (no warring or violence; complete pacifism), living a life of virtue, service to others, angelic assistance, spiritual communion and communal living when it is feasible to do so. Freedom and responsibility are two themes reiterated throughout the text of Oahspe.

And So...

If your present religion condones eating animals and you are concerned you may offend your church if you decide to pursue a vegetarian path, it's definitely time for a new spiritual approach in your life. You alone, have the right to choose, you have freedom of choice, above all…!

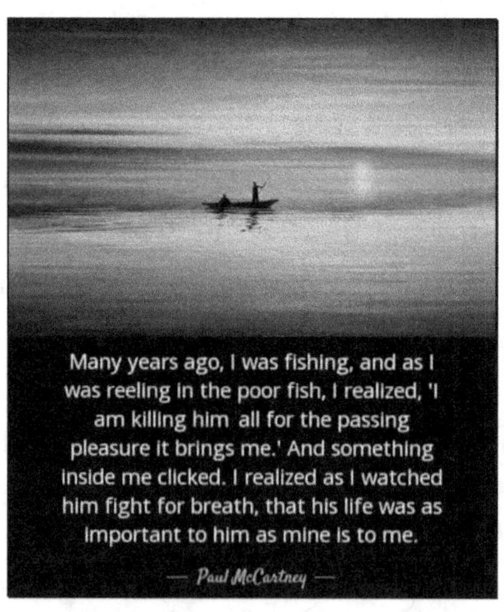

'The more I get to know humans, the more I prefer animals'

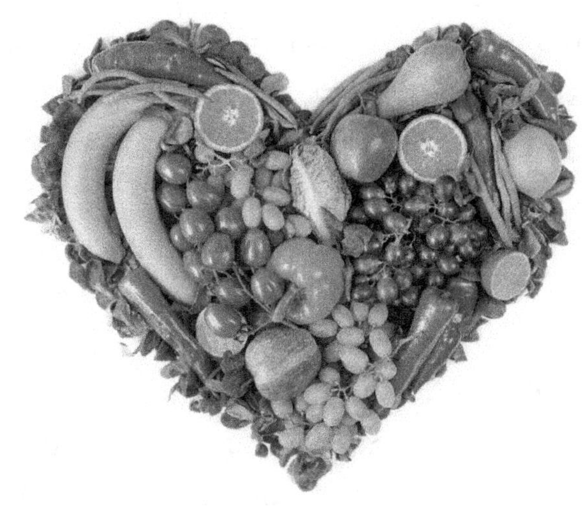

Plant- Based Foods

'Vegan is pure love'

Some say, plant-based diets are limited and bland. This is far from the truth. There are so many delicious vegan recipes and dishes available today, throughout the world, with mouth-watering flavours. Changing your diet to more plant-based meals, is a great way to induce a positive impact for climate change and biodiversity.

To take it a meaningful step further, we need to assert pressure on the companies producing nutrition to provide more wholesome, affordable plant-based foods, thereby reducing the amount of animal products available on shop shelves. This is a winner…!

There are many nutritious meat alternatives commercially available today, from burgers to sausages, mince and even cheese, with little difference in the taste or look. Meat substitutes are available in chicken, turkey, beef and pork flavours, made from soya, corn and various healthy whole grain ingredients, making it completely unnecessary to feast on innocent animals.

As previously mentioned, consuming the right food is crucial to maintaining a strong, healthy body. We tend to choose foods that are commercial rather than selecting foods that are healthy for us and this is where the bad habits begin.

One must be conscious in the moment and learn to listen to the body, which initially takes a bit of effort. Listening to the body is a matter of feeling it within. It sounds a little wacky but if you get into a routine of listening to your body, getting in tune with the respective vibrations of your body, it resonates quite naturally. Alternatively, if something doesn't taste good, let it go. This is your body telling you, warning you.

One must also take note of how the body responds to certain foods. Discomfort, feeling low, constipated, diarrhoea, agitated or nauseated after eating, is more than likely a sign, the body is being challenged. You also need to take cognisance of your food allergies. Don't aggravate them. Your body has an inherent intelligence. Every cell within your body is ingenious in its form and function with a complete blueprint requirement in order to function correctly and maintain a healthy physical structure.

'Real Food is Grown – not Born'

Eating is a wonderful and necessary preoccupation. Most people do it three times a day. Some people do it all day, it becomes an obsession. The objective of this chapter is not to chasten you but rather to show how you can live a healthy life from a plant-based diet, proving to you, there is no need to feast on innocent animals.

If you're carrying excess weight, a plant-based diet will trim you down fairly quickly. Plus, it will stabilise your sugar levels and get your heart rate back to healthy levels.

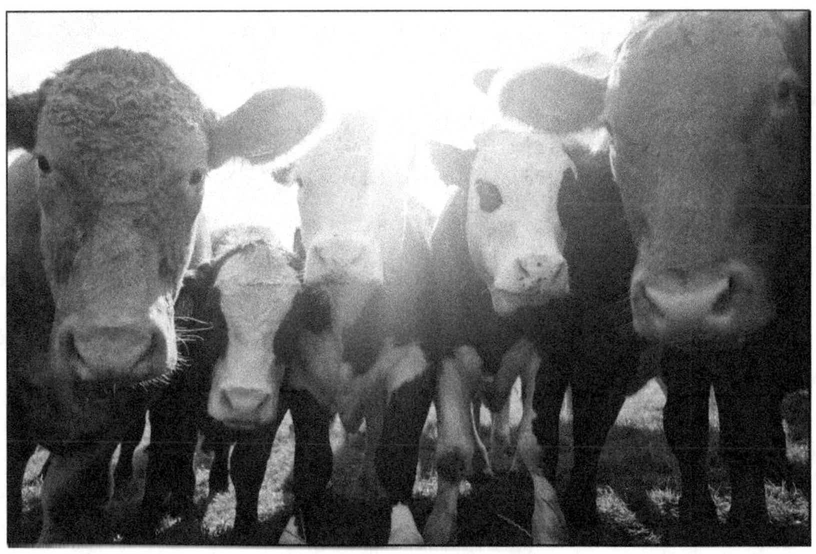

'Please don't eat me...!'

Initially, you will need to go on a complete three-day

detox program, consuming fruits and liquids only. Yes, it will be difficult. At times, you'll feel weak and even light headed. Mentally, you'll only be thinking about food. This is normal. Be strong, get through this detoxing period because it will be worth it. After the three-day period, your body will adjust. Your stomach will have shrunk a bit and adjusted, your bowels and bladder will slow down after a rather hectic period and mentally, you'll feel relaxed, clean and confident. The bonus is when you get on the bathroom scale and see how much weight you've lost…!

Your first introduction to real food after your fasting is a vegetable and fruit smoothie for breakfast. You will need a good liquidiser. The suggestion is as follows: Broccoli, Cabbage, Spinach and a carrot – take a small handful of each and dice it all up finely with a sharp knife on a board. Throw it all into your liquidiser jar. Next up is the fruit – preferably a banana or papaya (paw paw), plus an apple and a pear or two apples or whatever fruit selection you have available. Normally three fruits are sufficient – banana, apple and a pear. Dice them all up and throw them into the liquidiser. You should now have approximately an equal measure of fruit to vegetable mix. Add a piece of raw ginger (about half the size of your thumb) and squeeze a lemon (has so many good qualities…!) into your mix. This is your basic smoothie for every morning.

You can get creative by adding small amounts of nuts and raisins, cranberries, blueberries, etc. Plus, you can add any of the organic *'Superfoods'* available in the health sections of supermarkets or in Health Stores. The most popular are – concentrated greens in a powder form; alkaline powder (good for acid reduction); and calcium powder (good for strengthening bones, nails, hair, etc.). Add water to the jar and liquidise everything. You don't
want it too watery so don't overdo the water. Keep your blend to a nice firm mix.

It will be green in colour from the veggies but don't stress re the sight of it because it actually tastes okay. It's not going to win any prizes for taste but once you start drinking it, you get used to it fairly quickly. It's not exactly unpleasant to consume. Drink a glass full every hour or so and get it all down. If you down it all at once, all you're going to do is overload your kidneys, which you should always avoid, no matter what it is you're eating or drinking.

When it comes to your kidneys, moderation is key for these sensitive organs to operate efficiently. It's your kidneys that initially face the full attack when you bombard your system with cumbersome animal flesh, dairy, sugar overloads, pastries, alcohol, nicotine, etc., which create havoc on your sensitive digestion process because these toxic entities are perceived as invaders, often causing Acidosis (a condition in which kidneys fail to eliminate acid fast enough), including a whole host of other irksome problems.

Initially, you'll be consuming smoothies every day, Monday to Friday for breakfast for the next few months. Once your system adjusts and accepts this, you can reduce the smoothies to three times a week. However, you may not want to…!

On Saturday, have a break from smoothies and enjoy a bowl of Muesli or oats or bran flakes – nothing cooked and no sugared cereals…! On Sunday, you're back to fasting and this happens every Sunday – fruits and liquids only, all day.

Why do we do this…? It's because after a full night's sleep, your body's system is actually detoxing automatically. Now, when you wake up, your body needs to continue with its night's work and release all the unwanted toxins and matter. If you consume a fatty cooked breakfast when you wake up in the morning, you'll immediately clog up your system again instead of assisting the body's natural detox flow, which a raw fruit and veg smoothie will do, while still ensuring you receive healthy vitamins, minerals, natural proteins and carbs to carry you through to lunchtime.

Mondays to Saturdays for lunch – you can enjoy a couple of slices of Rye Bread (preferably avoid commercial breads), Rice Cakes, Crackers (preferably whole wheat). Basically, healthy substitutes for bread. For fillings on Rye bread/Crackers/Rice Cakes, etc., you can have bean or nut or chickpea salads or avocado, or even your favourite jams/toppings. Get creative, use the previous night's leftover curry, etc. Pasta salads are also awesome because of the carbs.

Dinner, is your first hot meal of the day. Always try and eat before 6:00pm because you need at least three to four hours of digestion time before you go to sleep at night, otherwise you'll be tossing and turning the whole night instead of sleeping.

Dinner should ideally, consist of a mix or vegetables (preferably raw, except pumpkin, potatoes, butternut, etc.), proteins, some carbs and a salad. The exact split between these four depends largely on what kind of daily activities you're currently undertaking. If it's a lot of hard physical work then obviously you need to increase your protein intake. If it's a long enduring day, you need more carbs and so on.

Plant-based proteins can be sourced from a variety of foods like legumes, nuts (especially almonds), seeds, whole grains, Tofu, Soya, beans, lentils, chick peas, etc. You can certainly get enough proteins by ensuring you consume one or two of these protein sources with every meal and even snacks, if possible.

With regards to snacks, we all love snacks...! The obvious choice is commercial health bars but caution needs to be applied here because some of the brands available on your supermarket shelf contain a lot of sugar (as much as 15gram per 100gram content), plus Whey powder and milk powders. Rather opt for a handful of sunflower seeds or mixed nuts as a heathier alternative. With fruits, a banana or an apple is really good and for veggies, a carrot is always an awesome healthy snack.

The graph line of protein intake goes up when it comes to athletic trainings. A lot of athlete's drool over animal protein sources for those bigger, toned muscles. However, swapping to plant-based proteins certainly helps performance and play, better than ever before. This is because plant-based proteins not only assist with better athletic performance but also with energy levels and especially, recovery time, which is vitally important.

In fact, the more one consumes plant proteins, the healthier the gut will be. This is due to the higher fibre content and nutritive value. Plant-based proteins help detox the overall body for this is how they fight off bodily infections. Plant based proteins, along with your natural protein levels, boost up the antioxidant levels as well. Antioxidants assist in the fight against free radicals, which cause aging. Healthy, glowing and supple skin is proportional to your plant foods intake.

Plant-Based Meat Alternatives...

A meat alternative or meat substitute is a food product made from vegetarian or vegan ingredients, eaten as a replacement for meat. Meat alternatives are engineered to mirror specific types of meat, such as mouth feel, flavour, appearance and even chemical characteristics.

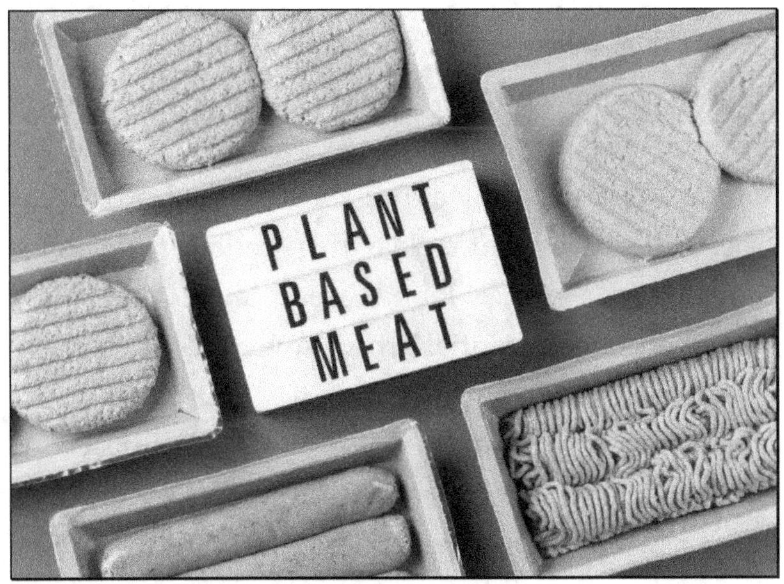

So Many Options...!

Plant-based meat has taken the healthy-eating world by storm. What was once a category reserved for rubbery soya-based sausage and chewy fake chicken nuggets is now a category, offering up some pretty impressive-tasting food. Plant-based meat may look and taste like your favourite meats but it's made from a variety of meat-free ingredients, like soya, pea, wheat gluten, pulses or even jackfruit. Some plant-based meats include salt, artificial colours, flavours and processing aids to generate a *'meat-like'* sensory appeal, so make sure you read the ingredients. Plant-based bacon, meatballs and other plant-based meats have a similar flavour, texture and appearance as the animal meat version, but without any animal-product content.

While a large percentage of people choose to eat plant-based meats for animal welfare or environmental reasons, many people choose these protein sources because it's healthier than eating a piece of chicken, steak or other meat. Regardless of a person's motivation to eat these meat alternatives, it's clear this trend is not going away any time soon. Plant-based meat markets have experienced substantial growth over recent years.

If you've been advised to limit your intake of processed meats, red meat or any animal-based product, for detrimental health reasons by your Doctor, then plant-based meats offer a natural solution, allowing people to enjoy their favourite foods, while complying with their health recommendations. Data published in 2018 in *Public Health Nutrition*, shows health benefits to eating less meat and replacing it with simple plant-based protein sources, like legumes and tofu, decreases a person's risk of developing cardiovascular disease, diabetes and certain cancers.

According to a study published in 2021 in *Nutrients*, before plant-based meat alternatives were available, those who chose to eat less meat and opt for more plant-based protein choices, included single-ingredient foods like tofu, lentils and nuts. The resulting dishes prepared were made with minimal oil and salt whereas, some plant-based meat options today, contain *'filler ingredients'*, which can potentially lead to a higher calorie, fat and salt intake.

Unlike those following a diet replacing meat with plant-based meats, those who replaced meat with plant-based protein sources like beans, legumes and nuts, met all daily micronutrient requirements.

If you enjoy plant-based meat alternatives and you want to continue including them in your diet, here are some tips to consider:

1. Enjoy plant-based meats as a part of a balanced diet that includes other protein sources, like legumes, nuts and seeds

2. Consider supplementation of key nutrients, like vitamin B12, if you are avoiding other protein sources

3. Opt for plant-based meat choices that are low in saturated fat and sodium

4. Eat plant-based meats with healthy foods and drinks, like whole grains and vegetables

Plant-based meats can be a healthy part of a balanced diet if you enjoy them in the right way. Consuming plant-based meats in moderation, along with fruits, veggies and other nutrient-dense foods, will profoundly support your health. However, only eating plant-based bacon, sausage and hot dogs as your protein source and avoiding choices like legumes, seeds, nuts and whole grains, is not a path to support the healthy outcomes you may want to achieve.

The best meals with the optimum results are often the more simple meals like – Lentil or a mixed bean curry with brown rice and diced veg; a lentil or mixed bean and brown rice stew; a mixed bean salad; hamburger patties, made from lentils or mixed beans (no eggs); a lentil cottage pie with mashed potato; chickpeas and pasta dishes (there are so many you can do); Samp and Beans (a staple diet in Africa); the list of combos you can do, is in fact endless.

The more you get into cooking in a healthy way, the quicker you'll begin creating your own special recipes. It's pointless providing a set of recipes for this book because all you need do is Google – *'Vegan Recipes'* – and you will get hundreds of awesome, scrumptious tried and trusted recipes, catering for all your needs and food desires.

Be healthy, be positive and live a good wholesome life, free of guilt re the needless slaughter of innocent animal life, which is so unnecessary…!

Plant-Based Proteins

The following is a list of the finer plant-based proteins readily available:

Seitan

Seitan is a popular protein source, made from gluten, which is the main protein in wheat. Unlike many soy-based mock meats, it closely resembles the look and texture of meat when cooked. It's also referred to as *'Wheat Meat'* or

'Wheat Gluten'. The protein ratio is very high at 25 grams of protein per 100 grams, making it one of the richest plant protein sources available. Seitan is also a good source of selenium and it contains small amounts of iron, calcium, and phosphorus. You can find this meat alternative in the refrigerated section of many grocery stores, especially in health food stores. You can also make your own version with Vital wheat gluten. Seitan can be pan-fried, sautéed or grilled, making it easy to incorporate into a variety of recipes. However, because it contains wheat, people with gluten-related disorders should avoid eating Seitan.

Tofu, Tempeh and Edamame

Tofu, Tempeh and Edamame, all originate from soybeans. They are especially popular in East Asian cuisine. Soybeans are considered a whole source of protein, meaning they provide all the essential amino acids the body requires. Edamame are immature soybeans with a sweet and slightly grassy taste. They need to be steamed or boiled prior to consumption. They can be enjoyed on their own or added to soups, salads, sushi, wraps, stir-fries, or rice rolls. Tofu is made from bean curds pressed together in a process similar to cheesemaking. Meanwhile, Tempeh is made by cooking and slightly fermenting mature soybeans, before pressing them into a block. Tofu doesn't have much taste on its own, but it easily absorbs the flavour of the ingredients it's prepared with. Comparatively, Tempeh has a characteristic nutty flavour. Both Tofu and Tempeh can be used in a variety of recipes, ranging from burgers to soups, stews, curries and chilis.

These three soy-based proteins contain iron, calcium and 12/20 grams of protein per 100-gram serving. Edamame is also rich in folate, vitamin K and fibre, which helps support digestion and bowel regularity. Tempeh contains probiotics, B vitamins and minerals such as magnesium and phosphorus.

Lentils

With 18 grams of protein per cooked cup (198 grams), lentils are a great source of protein. They can be used in a variety of dishes, ranging from fresh salads to hearty soups, stews and spice-infused dahls. Lentils are also a great source of fibre, providing over half of the daily recommended fibre intake in a single cup (198 grams). Furthermore, the type of fibre found in lentils, feeds the good bacteria in the colon, which helps promote a healthy gut. Lentils also reduce the chance of heart disease, diabetes, excess body weight and certain types of cancer. In addition, lentils are rich in folate, manganese and iron. They also contain a hearty dose of antioxidants and other health-promoting plant compounds. You can use lentils in a variety of recipes, ranging from cottage pies and curries to veggie burgers. Lentils are popular around the globe. They are the basis of many Indian dishes. If you eat South Asian food often, chances are, you're already a huge fan of lentils.

Beans

Kidney, black, pinto, sugar, butter and most other varieties of beans are extremely important staple foods across cultures, containing high amounts of protein per serving. Beans are probably the most versatile protein form available. They exist in numerous dishes as fillers but are also the primary dish for many cultures globally. Chickpeas, also known as garbanzo beans, are another type of bean with a high protein content. Most types of beans contain about 15 grams of protein per cooked cup (170 grams). They're also excellent sources of complex carbs, fibre, iron, folate, phosphorus, potassium, manganese and several beneficial plant compounds. Moreover, several studies show, a diet rich in beans and other legumes helps decrease cholesterol levels, manages blood sugar, lowers blood pressure and even reduces belly fat. Add beans to your diet by making a tasty bowl of homemade chili, or enjoy extra health benefits by sprinkling a dash of turmeric on roasted chickpeas. Make bean stews, bean soups, bean casseroles, bean salads with pasta, bean burgers – the recipe range is indeed endless with this very versatile high protein source.

Nutritional Yeast

Nutritional yeast is a deactivated strain of Saccharomyces cerevisiae yeast, which is sold commercially as a yellow powder or flakes. It has a cheesy flavour, which makes it a popular ingredient in dishes like mashed potatoes and scrambled Tofu. Nutritional yeast can also be sprinkled on top of pasta dishes or even enjoyed as a savoury topping on popcorn. 16 grams of this complete source of plant protein provides 8 grams of protein and 3 grams of fibre. Fortified nutritional yeast is also an excellent source of zinc, magnesium, copper, manganese and all the B vitamins, including vitamin B12.

However, keep in mind, not all types of nutritional yeast are fortified, so be sure to check the label carefully, especially the fine print.

Spelt and Teff

Spelt and Teff belong to a category known as ancient grains. Other ancient grains include einkorn, barley, farro and sorghum. Spelt is a type of wheat, it contains gluten, whereas Teff originates from an annual grass, meaning its naturally gluten-free. Spelt and Teff provide 10/11 grams of protein per cooked cup (250 grams), making them higher in protein than other ancient grains. Both are excellent sources of various nutrients, including complex carbs, fibre, iron, magnesium, phosphorus and manganese. They also contain B vitamins, zinc and Selenium. Spelt and Teff are versatile alternatives to other grains, such as wheat and rice. They can be used in many recipes ranging from baked goods to risotto. In fact, flour made from Teff is the key ingredient in Injera, a flatbread commonly eaten in East Africa, such as in Ethiopia, Eritrea, and Sudan.

Hemp Seeds

Hemp seeds come from the Cannabis sativa plant, which is sometimes maligned for belonging to the same family as the cannabis plant. However, hemp seeds contain only minor trace amounts of tetrahydrocannabinol (THC), the compound that produces the psychoactive effects of cannabis. Although hemp seeds aren't as well-known as other seeds, they contain 9 grams of protein in each 3-tablespoon (30-gram) serving. Hemp seeds also contain high levels of magnesium, iron, calcium, zinc and selenium. What's more, they're a good source of omega-3 and omega-6 fatty acids in the ratio considered optimal for human health. Interestingly, some studies indicate, the type of fats found in hemp seeds reduce inflammation and alleviate symptoms of premenstrual syndrome, menopause and certain skin conditions. Add hemp seeds to your diet by sprinkling some in your smoothie or morning muesli. They can also be used in homemade salad dressings, granola, energy balls or protein bars. Who would have thought back in the 60's & 70's, people legally growing hemp and converting it to everything from food to fuel…!

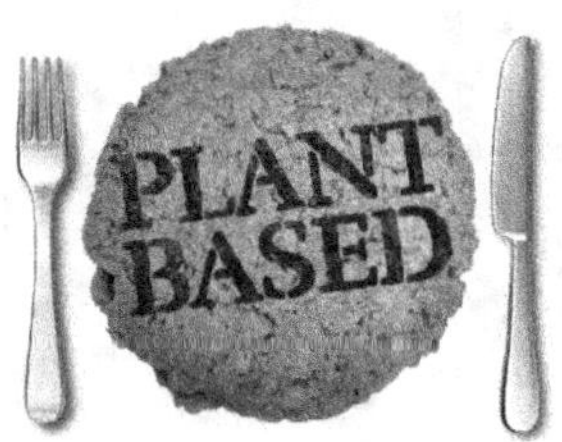

'Animals are here With us, not For us'

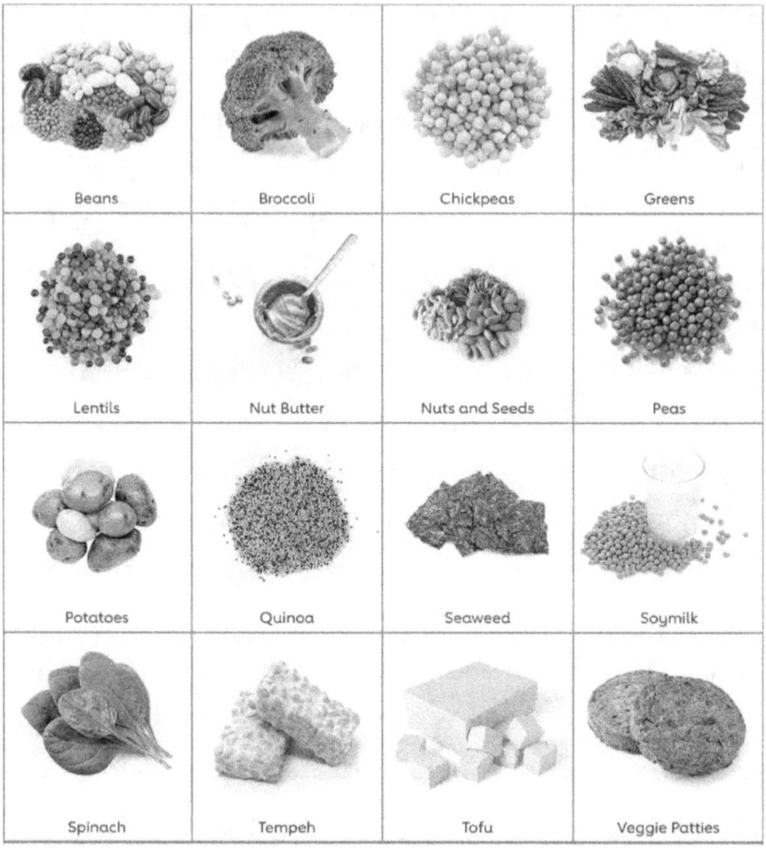

Beans	Broccoli	Chickpeas	Greens
Lentils	Nut Butter	Nuts and Seeds	Peas
Potatoes	Quinoa	Seaweed	Soymilk
Spinach	Tempeh	Tofu	Veggie Patties

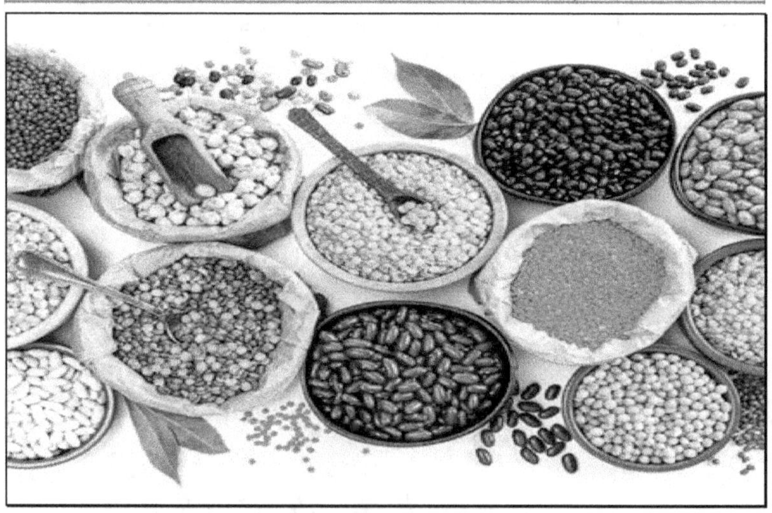

Green Peas

Green peas contain nearly 9 grams of protein per cooked cup (160 grams), which is slightly more than a cup (237 ml) of dairy milk. What's more, a serving of green peas covers more than 25% of your daily fibre, thiamine, folate, manganese and vitamin A, C, and K needs. Green peas are also a good source of iron, magnesium, phosphorus, zinc, copper and several other B vitamins. You can use peas in recipes such as pea-and-basil-stuffed ravioli, Thai-inspired pea soup or pea-and-avocado guacamole.

'All we are saying, is give peas a chance...!'

Amaranth and Quinoa

Although Amaranth and Quinoa are often referred to as ancient or gluten-free grains, they don't grow from grasses like other cereal grains do. For this reason, they're technically considered pseudo cereals. Nevertheless, similar to more commonly known grains, they can be prepared or ground into flours. Amaranth and Quinoa provide 8/9 grams of protein per cooked cup (185 grams) and are complete sources of protein, which is uncommon among grains and pseudo cereals. Plus, Amaranth and Quinoa are good sources of complex carbs, fibre, iron, manganese, phosphorus, and magnesium.

Spirulina

This blue-green alga, is definitely a nutritional powerhouse. A 14 gram serving provides 8 grams of complete protein, in addition to covering 22% of your daily requirements for iron and 95% of your daily copper needs. Spirulina also contains high amounts of magnesium, riboflavin, manganese, potassium and small amounts of other nutrients your body needs, including essential fatty acids. According to some test-tube studies, phycocyanin, a natural pigment found in spirulina, also appears to have powerful antioxidant, anti-inflammatory and anti-cancer properties. Studies also link spirulina to health benefits ranging from a stronger immune system and reduced blood pressure to improved blood sugar and cholesterol levels.

'Gram for gram, Spirulina could be the most nutritious and well-rounded food on the planet, which stores almost indefinitely' - Gabriel Cousens

Ezekiel Bread

Ezekiel bread is made from organic, sprouted whole grains and legumes. These include wheat, millet, barley and spelt, as well as soybeans and lentils. Two slices of Ezekiel bread contain approximately 8 grams of protein, which is slightly more than other types of bread. Sprouting grains and legumes increase the number of healthy nutrients. They contain and reduce the content of antinutrients, which are compounds, affecting the body's absorption of certain vitamins and minerals. In addition, studies show, sprouting increases their content of specific amino acids, such as lysine, which can help boost their overall protein quality.

Similarly, combining grains with legumes further improves the bread's amino acid profile. Sprouting also seems to boost the content of soluble fibre, folate, vitamins C and E and beta carotene. It also reduces gluten, which can improve digestion among people with gluten-related disorders.

Chia Seeds

Chia seeds are derived from the Salvia Hispanica plant, which is native to Mexico and Guatemala. With 5 grams of protein and 10 grams of fibre per 28 grams, Chia seeds definitely deserve their spot on the list of top plant-based proteins. These little seeds contain high levels of iron, calcium, Selenium and magnesium, as well as omega-3 fatty acids, antioxidants and other beneficial plant compounds. They're also incredibly versatile. Thanks to their mild taste and ability to absorb water, they form a gel-like substance. This quality makes them an easy addition for a variety of recipes, ranging from smoothies to baked goods and chia pudding.

Sunflower Seeds

Sunflower seeds are harvested from the flower head of the sunflower plant. While the seed itself is encased in a black and white striped shell, sunflower seeds are white and have a tender texture. Known for their distinct nutty flavour and high nutritional value, you can eat the seeds raw, roasted or incorporated into other dishes. Studies link the consumption of sunflower seeds to a number of health benefits, including lowering the risk of developing diseases like high blood pressure or heart disease. They also contain nutrients that support the immune system and boost energy levels.

For those with short-term or chronic inflammation, sunflower seeds can offer anti-inflammatory benefits. Sunflower seeds contain vitamin E, flavonoids and other plant compounds that reduce inflammation. A study found, consuming sunflower seeds and other seeds, five times or more each week resulted in lower levels of inflammation, which also lowers risk factors for several chronic diseases. Sunflower seeds are rich in *'healthy'* fats, including polyunsaturated fat and monounsaturated fat. A three-fourths cup serving of sunflower seeds contains 14 grams of fat. Studies found, consumption of sunflower seeds is linked to reduced rates of cardiovascular disease, high cholesterol and high blood pressure.

Sunflower seeds are a source of many vitamins and minerals that support your immune system and increase your ability to fight off viruses. These include both zinc and Selenium. Zinc plays a vital role in the immune system, helping the body maintain and develop immune cells. Selenium also plays a role in fighting infection, and boosting immunity.

While the high levels of protein in sunflower seeds already help boost energy levels, other nutrients like vitamin B and Selenium keep one energized. The vitamin B1 (also known as Thiamine) present in sunflower seeds, helps convert food to energy, keeping one active throughout the day. Selenium increases blood flow and delivers more oxygen to the body.

Sunflower seeds are high in protein and rich in healthy fats, as well as antioxidants. They are an excellent source of: Vitamin E; Vitamin B1; Vitamin B6; Iron; Copper; Selenium; Manganese; Zinc; and Potassium. According to the **USDA**, ¼ cup of dry roasted sunflower seeds without salt contains: Calories - 207; Protein - 5.8 grams; Fat - 19 grams; Carbohydrates - 7 grams; and Fibre - 3.9 grams.

Sunflower seeds are typically consumed in a variety of dishes - sprinkle on top of a salad; add to a trail mix; stir into oatmeal; sprinkle over stir fry or mixed vegetables; add to veggie burgers; mix into baked goods. Preferably, use sunflower butter in place of peanut butter and cook with sunflower oil instead of other oils.

'Don't judge each other by the harvest you reap, rather by the seeds you plant' – Robert Louis Stevenson

Nuts, Nut Butters & Other Seeds

Nuts, seeds and their derived products are great sources of protein. Every 28 grams contains 5/7 grams of protein, depending on the variety. Nuts and seeds are also great sources of fibre and healthy fats, along with iron, calcium, magnesium, selenium, phosphorus, vitamin E and certain B vitamins. They likewise contain antioxidants, among other beneficial plant compounds. When choosing which nuts and seeds to buy, keep in mind, blanching and roasting may damage the nutrients in nuts. Therefore, best to select raw, unblanched versions whenever possible. Also, try opting for natural nut butters to avoid the oil, sugar and excess salt, which is often added to many popular brands.

Oats and Oatmeal

Eating oats is an easy and delicious way to add protein to any diet. Half a cup (40 grams) of dry oats provides approximately 5 grams of protein and 4 grams of fibre. Oats also contain magnesium, zinc, phosphorus and folate. Although oats are not considered a complete protein, they do contain a higher quality protein than other commonly consumed grains compared to rice and wheat. You can use oats in a variety of recipes ranging from oatmeal to veggie burgers. They can also be ground into flour and used for baking.

Wild Rice & Brown Rice

Both types of rice are great sources of fibre, antioxidants and nutrients like manganese, magnesium, copper and phosphorus. However, Brown rice contains more B vitamins compared to Wild rice, making it a great choice if you're on a meat-free diet. Wild rice contains more protein than regular rice and many other grains. A 100-gram serving of Wild rice provides 4 grams of protein, which is twice as much as regular rice and approximately 1.5 times more than other long-grain rice varieties, like Basmati. Unlike white rice, wild rice is not stripped of its bran, which is great from a nutritional perspective, as bran contains fibre and plenty of vitamins and minerals.

Alternative Milks...

There are many popular milk alternatives available on the open market such as Soy milk; Oat Milk; Almond Milk; Coconut Milk; Macadamia Milk and so on...

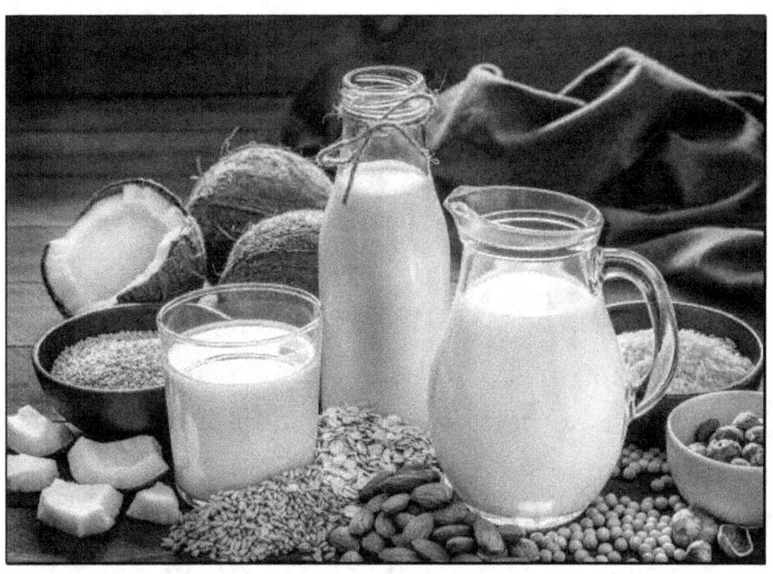

Soy Milk...

Made from soybeans, usually fortified with vitamins and

minerals. It can be a great alternative to dairy milk for those who avoid dairy for allergic reasons. Not only does it contain 6 grams of protein per cup (244 ml), it's also an excellent source of vitamin A and B plus Potassium, Calcium, Retinol, Folate and Choline. You can purchase soy milk in most supermarkets. It's an incredibly versatile product. Can be consumed independently or used in a variety of cooking and baking recipes. Some Soy blends may contain added sugar. For weight control, preferably opt for unsweetened varieties whenever possible. Soy milk is often used by infants who suffer from dairy allergies.

Oat Milk...

Oat milk is simply rolled oats and water blended together then strained to leave the pulp behind. The result is easy, creamy oat milk. Nutrients from the oats remain in the milk. The fine particles give the liquid a creamy texture. Unflavoured oat milk retains a faint oat flavour.

Almond Milk...

Almond milk is made by blending almonds with water and then straining the mixture to remove the solids. You can also make it by adding water to almond butter. It has a pleasant, nutty flavour and a creamy texture similar to cow's milk. For this reason, it is a popular choice for those who are allergic or intolerant to dairy. Commercial almond milk is available in a variety of brands and scrumptious flavours. For health reasons, it is best to choose unsweetened almond milk. Almond milk contains many minerals and vitamins, especially vitamin E and D. It's also low in calories with one cup of almond milk containing only 39 calories, which is half the number of calories in a cup of skim dairy milk.

Macadamia Milk...

Like most other plant-based milk, macadamia milk is made by soaking the raw nuts in water for several hours before blending to a puree and filtered to produce the final healthy and nutritious drink. Macadamia nuts are usually blended with filtered/treated water, salt, plus additional flavourings as required, such as cocoa powder, fruit or dates, to sweeten the milk. The result is creamy, fresh macadamia milk, perfect for Matcha Lattes, Golden milk and even baked goods like muffins or cookies. Macadamia milk has fewer calories and less sugar than cow's milk, with similar levels of calcium and vitamin D. It is one of the lowest carb options for plant-based milk and it's typically free of Carrageenan, which is a substance extracted from red and purple seaweeds, used as a thickening or emulsifying agent in food products.

'Macadamia Milk promotes healthy hair growth...!'

Coconut Milk...

Coconut milk is an opaque, white liquid extracted from the meat of a mature coconut. The traditional method for making coconut milk involves grating coconut flesh, mixing it with hot water and pressing the liquid through cheesecloth, traditionally working it by hand. This process produces a rich, fatty liquid known as coconut cream. Coconut cream can be further processed into coconut oil or pressed again to make coconut milk. With little or no water added, rich coconut cream is obtained. Whereas, adding water and greater working produces thinner milk. Commercially processed coconut milk, is grated and pressed mechanically, often stabilised with the addition of Guar gum. Coconut milk has fewer nutrients than dairy milk. While many brands of coconut milk provide calcium, vitamin A, vitamin B12 and vitamin D, these nutrients are mostly fortified. Be aware - just because coconut products don't contain animal-derived ingredients, it doesn't always mean they don't cause harm. As the investigation into the Thai coconut industry revealed, monkeys may be abused and exploited for coconut picking so that these products can end up on our shelves.

Protein-Rich Fruits & Vegetables

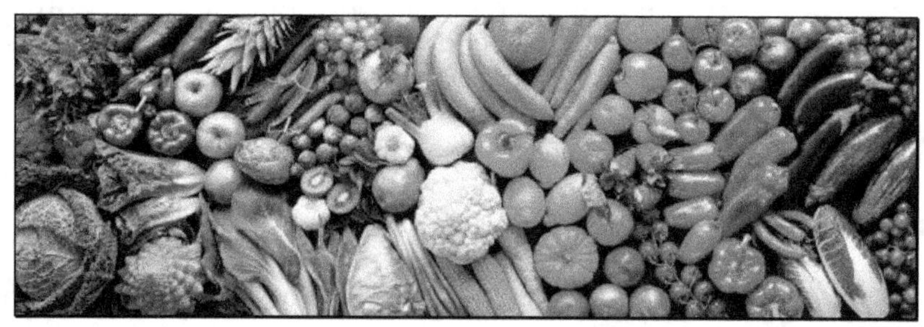

Although all fruits and vegetables contain protein, some

obviously contain more than others. Vegetables with the most protein include broccoli, spinach, asparagus, artichokes, potatoes, sweet potatoes and Brussel sprouts, which typically contain 4/5 grams of protein per cooked cup. Sweet corn is another common food, containing a similar protein count as other high protein vegetables. Fresh fruits generally have a lower protein content than vegetables. Those containing the most protein include: guava, cherimoyas, mulberries, blackberries, nectarines and bananas, which have about 2/4 grams of protein per cup. For balance, you should try and consume at least five vegetables and equally, five fruits every day.

Mycoprotein

Mycoprotein is a non-animal-based protein derived from Fusarium Venanatin, which is a type of fungus. It's often used to produce meat substitutes, including veggie burgers, patties, cutlets and fillets. The nutritional value can range a bit depending on the specific product. Most contain 15/16 grams of protein per 100gram serving, along with 5/8 grams of fibre. Although there were concerns once related to food allergies, research shows adverse reactions are rare. However, keep in mind, some products made with Mycoprotein may also contain egg whites, so be sure to check the label carefully if you're following a vegan diet or avoiding eggs for other reasons, such as food allergies.

'Fifty percent of the weight of a soybean is protein'

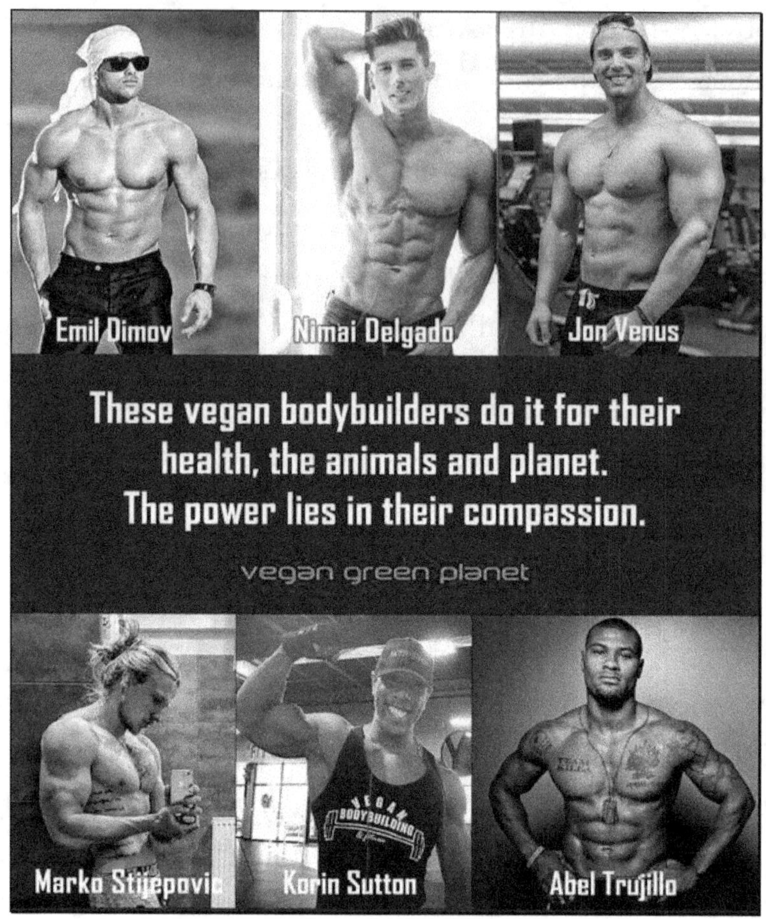

And So...

Including a protein-rich ingredient in each meal or snack is a great way to boost your protein intake. Try topping salads with Tofu, sprinkling nutritional yeast over popcorn or pairing fresh fruit with nut butter to squeeze some extra protein into your diet. There's so much you can do. Go out and experiment, create your own recipes and have fun…!

Nowadays, protein deficiencies among vegetarians and vegan followers are rare, especially those on a dedicated health path, because they usually follow a well-planned diet and maintain it. Years ago, we didn't have the science or availability re the many easy access protein food sources we have today. There really is no excuse not to live a healthier lifestyle in this modern age of easy entrée to natural foods.

There are many reasons folk desire to live a plant-based diet. Some commit to it for the natural health it offers in comparison to a burdening flesh and blood diet, which has an even chance of inducing cancer, a heart attack or a stroke at some time in their life. Others do it to maintain a trim and enhanced physique. And then there are those who love animals and have absolutely no desire to consume an innocent animal. Finally, a lot of folk do it for religious reasons. Whatever your reason, we all need to learn to respect all life because all life is ultimately precious. Our planet is very special and needs to be shared with all species mutually.

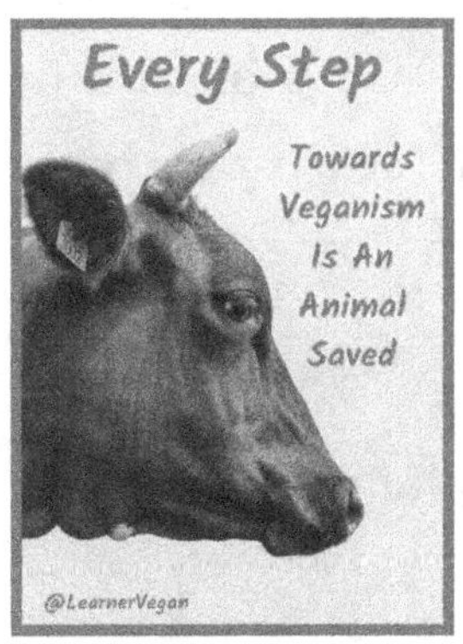

Feel the beets, lose the meats, go vegan' – Jermaine Dupri

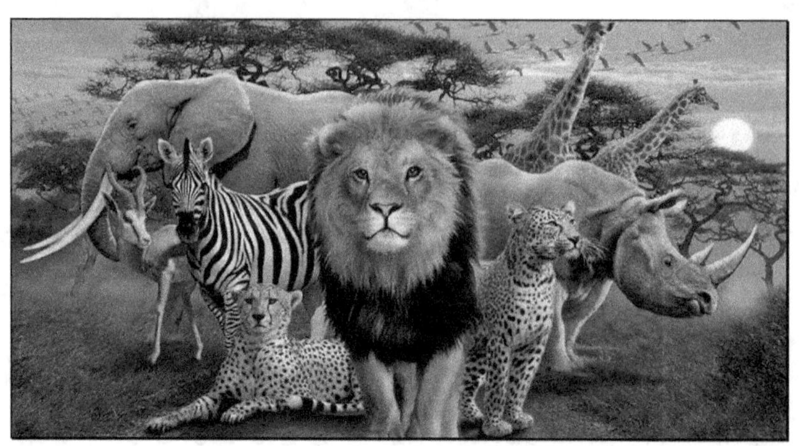

Extinction & Other Nasties...

'Animals are innocent sufferers in a hell of our making'
Jeffrey Moussaieff Masson

Sadly, there are numerous animals facing extinction globally, many are on the critical list. Man's massive, destructive footprint has driven countless animals to extinction already. We look at a few of the larger species facing a perilous future but first we home in on some disturbing facts on domestic animal treatment for human consumption…

1.) Dairy Industry

The dairy industry is a global, shocking horror story. Calves are removed from their mothers at birth so farmers can milk the bloated mother cows, knowing full well, cow milk is suitable for calves and absolutely not suitable for humans. The dairy industry likes to inform consumers, a glass of milk is the perfect drink, even for athletes who need to recover, because it contains carbohydrates, protein and fat.

And it's true, for a baby cow, milk is a nutrient-dense drink. However, when humans drink it, we get a nasty cocktail of saturated fat, testosterone, oestrogen, trans fat and many other evils, especially allergy evils. Our defence mechanisms detect this food source as an invader and immediately create internal antibodies to fight it, which causes inflammation. Inflammation is the great inhibitor of repair and recovery for the human body, in particular, athletes. Sadly, for most of us, inflammation is also the impetus to chronic diseases. In addition, it's well known and documented, farmers pump cows with huge doses of antibiotics, hormone stimulants and whatever else they can, to accelerate growth in the animals and help fight infection. These detrimental drugs are then passed onto humans via drinking the milk and eating the flesh.

It's a complete no-win situation, neither for humans or especially for the innocent cows. Cow milk is rated as one of the most disease driven foods consumed by humans. Milk curdles in one's stomach, creating harmful digestive disorders, with major compounding effects on the remainder of the system. Cow's milk should have been banned eons ago. There are so many nourishing alternative milk products available today, like Almond and Soya milk, making the need for cow's milk redundant. To steal a mother's calf at birth is unthinkable. The cows bellow for days on end in search of their beloved calves. Imagine doing that to human mothers.

The constant neglect, horrific cruelty and abuse from mankind on the planet's animals are at times unthinkable. It is without doubt one of the largest drawbacks for man's spiritual development on earth. Until such time as we come to terms with this and actively do something about it, the world will continue to suffer as a consequence.

2.) Poultry Industry

The chicken industry is also sickening. Raising chickens for their eggs isn't as wholesome a practice as the egg industry wants you to believe. In fact, the suffering and mistreatment of layer hens make it one of the cruellest types of farming in the food industry. Whether they're raised to lay eggs or for their meat, chickens in factory farming operations suffer needless cruelty and vile death methods. *PETA* calls chickens 'the most abused animals on the planet.' They the most-slain animals for the purposes of feeding humans, more chickens are killed for food every year than all other land animals combined.

Poultry farming disrupts the family unit among chickens, denying the birds their needs for social interactions and good nutrition, forcing them into cruel conditions until they're inhumanely slaughtered. And all because people can't get enough eggs, fried chicken, baked chicken, chicken casserole, chicken salad, etc. If humans gave up these foods and replaced them with plant-based substitutes, chickens wouldn't have to face the cruel realities of poultry farming.

Many people believe layer hens aren't treated poorly because they're not killed for meat. The reality is, they're given no more room or mercy than birds raised for meat. Chickens aren't allowed to nest, or to care for their young. Layer hens are housed in extremely cramped conditions with no access to sunlight. Furthermore, they're bred specifically for speed laying, increasing egg production per hen. Since they're not biologically designed to lay that many eggs, they suffer painful health problems, which are passed on to the human consumer.

When farmers raise animals for the sole purpose of killing them, they disrupt the ecosystem and deny animals their rights. Chickens lay eggs for the purpose of giving birth to healthy chicks. When farmers steal eggs from chickens, they deny them the opportunity to naturally propagate their species. Worse, farmers hasten the breeding of chickens for human consumption, consuming resources like grain in staggering quantities. All animals have inbred behaviours that serve very specific purposes. Many birds, including chickens, give themselves dust baths. They move around in dry dirt, dust, or sand to remove contaminants, such as parasites, from their feathers and skin. Dust baths are also a chicken's natural way of marking their territory. They leave pheromones behind to tell other chickens where they've been. Poultry farming doesn't allow chickens to engage in dust baths. They're unable to clean themselves, which means they suffer infections of the skin and feathers as well as immeasurable frustration. They will never get to build a nest, which is in their genes. They don't get to stretch their legs, peck the ground looking for grubs, or participate in any other behaviour to which chickens instinctively gravitate.

To cram more chickens into small spaces, poultry farms use vertical battery cages, like live animals kept in the despicable Chinese wet markets. The wire bottoms don't give layer hens a comfortable place to roost or stand. Since battery cages have wire bottoms, faeces and urine fall from the top cages into the bottom cages. This is particularly harmful to the layer hens on the bottom of the stack as the faeces and urine are caught in the feathers of the chickens directly below. Bacteria cultivates and causes disease. The ammonia from urine causes burned eyes, ears and nasal passages as well as throat discomfort. This sadly sets in motion a series of injurious diseases. When chickens contract salmonella prior to being slaughtered, the disease is passed on to the human consumer. Symptoms of salmonella poisoning, include digestive discomfort, nausea, vomiting, diarrhoea and fever.

Since male chicks can't lay eggs, they're slaughtered immediately after birth. The wholesale destruction of zillions of male chicks involves gassing, boiling and grinding while the innocent chicks are still alive. These tiny, innocent birds aren't even granted a humane death. Their only crime – they were born on God's earth. Shame on mankind for allowing this to happen…!

Layer and broiler hens are bred to reach maturity in a matter of days rather than months. Through genetic mutations, hormone injections and other distorted cocktails, the birds reach puberty far earlier than nature intended. However, their tiny little bodies weren't designed to support the advanced weight gains experienced from these genetic mutations, so the extra weight gained at a very tender age, stresses their bones and joints. Because of this, many go lame long before they're slaughtered. Some develop deformities of the legs and wings. They end their short, bitter lives in extreme pain with no veterinary care because their only purpose is to provide meat for humans. How sick is this industry…?

'We need so little in life and yet we ask for so much'
- Kiko Michel –

3.) Elephants...

Elephants are everyone's favourite animal. They have deep emotions plus they're extremely family orientated. If you do a game walk and observe elephants, you'll get to learn a bit about them. They're either left or right-handed, respond to love like a dog, are very playful, sometimes even cheeky.

They have a mischievous sense of humour, are very sensitive, quick to anger if upset and will defend their herd to the death when threatened. They have amazing memories, grieve like humans over the loss of a herd member, display incredible mothering skills and have a deep cognitive and emotional intelligence.

There is a famous elephant in Taiwan called *'SUDA'*. She paints self-portraits of herself in stick form and even signs her name. You can call it up on You Tube, lovely to witness. It takes an entire elephant herd to raise just one calf. They all care for the little ones because gestation takes almost two years, so their young are very precious. A single herd is led by a Matriarch. There is strict order. The herd is a tight cohesive unit. Man is not easily accepted in their environment, considering humans hunt/poach, steal their young for zoos/circuses and private Game Parks, etc., illegally export their ivory to China and the eastern countries and so on. It is despicable what mankind has done and is still doing to these magnificent animals who display deeper social emotions than even humans.

Elephants are the real *'kings'* in the animal world. They have no predators other than man and occasionally lions, who will attack an isolated sick or old elephant or they'll prey on unprotected young calves. Elephants eventually die at around sixty to seventy years old when their teeth fall out and they can no longer eat. They are the most amazing animals with an abundance of beautiful energy.

Sadly, their numbers are dwindling at a rapid rate as demand from the east for their ivory increases. Ruthless poachers are quick to respond for financial gain throughout Africa. Around 40,000 elephants are murdered every year. It is difficult to comprehend how any sensible human could be a part of this terrible slaughter. If you feel the need to get involved then please log onto any of the many elephant sites for anti-poaching, donations, welfare, rehabilitation centres, etc.

The late *Lawrence Anthony*, who owned a Game Reserve in South Africa, was known as *'The Elephant Whisperer'*, a title he earned when he saved two elephant herds destined for culling because of farm destruction they had caused. At his own expense, Anthony transported the herds to his private Game Reserve in Zululand and cared for them. Initially the Matriarch of the herds wanted nothing to do with him but eventually accepted this passionate human and welcomed him into the herd.

Years later when Lawrence Anthony died, both herds travelled from their far away locations, through the wild Zululand veldt to Anthony's house. Neither of the herds had been near his house for over a year. Back in the day, the herds used to raid his garden and drink from his swimming pool. Both herds took up sentry at the garden wall of the house and stayed for two days in silent respect for this great man who had done so much for them. None of the local wildlife experts could explain how the elephants knew Anthony had passed away.

If we are God's caretakers of Mother Earth then we need to make a globally concerted effort to protect our wildlife, all of our wildlife, especially Africa's elephants and rhinos because with man's insatiable greed, there won't be any left in the near future.

If you visit Africa, experience the real Africa, get down and get dirty. Smell that dry earth, listen to the raw, poignant cry of the fish eagle and witness the animals in their natural habitat. It's wild. Explore and you will find yourself. This is what going with the flow is all about. You'll feel so balanced and centred after an African experience. Definitely good medicine…!

4.) Dolphins

Each year over 100,000 dolphins and small whales are killed in hunts across the globe. While the hunts taking place in Japan and the Faroe Islands are well documented, hunts take place in other parts of the world on almost a daily basis. Since 1990, people in at least 114 countries consumed one or more of at least 87 species of marine mammal. Yet only a few percent of the small whales, dolphins and porpoises actually consumed will ever be reported in official reports due to the illegality of the practice and the fact that much of the trade is therefore driven underground.

On an almost daily basis, numerous dolphin hunts are being undertaken in countries throughout West Africa, Latin America, the Caribbean, the South Pacific and Asia. The reasons for the hunts (which can include single or multiple individuals) vary from place to place with some claiming traditional and cultural beliefs. In some places, the availability of dolphin flesh originally stemmed from using dolphins who were unintentionally caught in fishing nets for bait and/or food. The practice has evolved both due to an acquired taste for the meat, as well as the inability to sustain families with food, as fish resources continue to plummet due to over-exploitation.

One year ago today, 1,423 Atlantic white-sided dolphins, including mothers with calves and pregnant females, were chased for hours before being murdered on a beach in the Faroe Islands. Death would not have come quickly. We can only imagine these highly intelligent and sensitive animals fear and confusion as they listened in vain to their pod mates' cries and screams before also suffering the pain and agony inflicted by the human knives, as they flayed the innocent animals alive in merciless cold blood. What kind of human stoops this low…?

A year later, despite international and domestic outrage

and public condemnation, little has changed. Shortly after the biggest hunt of dolphins in the islands' history, the Prime Minister announced a review of dolphin hunting in the Faroe Islands. Instead of a ban (which is something almost 60% of the Faroese public wanted, in particular - the *'Aquaculture Association'* and all its loyal members) an annual quota of 500 *'dolphins'* was given. This new quota is only in place until 2024 by which time it will be increased to 825. The announcement was nothing more than a slap in the face and a one-fingered salute to all those opposed to the hunting of dolphins. The review was an opportunity for the Faroe Islands to put to bed the needless slaughter of dolphins once and for all. Instead, it has further enshrined the killing of dolphins in national legislation.

Decisions were also made to further the development of a new *'dolphin killing tool'* and they offered a training course for the *'grind'* where participants are trained in the use of the new Spinal Lance (*sick*) for killing pilot whales. Sincerely hope they used humans as decoys for the training…just saying…

Let us not forget the butchering of six (protected) northern bottlenose whales over the course of a few days in August. It is illegal to hunt this species, but if the dolphins strand then they are allowed to be *'taken'*. However, it is the loose interpretation of *'strand'* that one must question as it's more like *'assisted stranding'* than anything else. None of this sounds as though there is any intention to ban, let alone reduce, dolphin hunting.

Dolphins (not including pilot whales, who are technically dolphins but not included in this review or included in the quotas set), are not seen as being a *'traditional hunt'* and as noted, plenty of Faroese people, including the fishing industry, wanted to see an end to these unnecessary and brutal killings. Dolphins were never a targeted species and individuals or pods were killed as and when they happened to be caught up in a pilot whale grind, as dolphins like to hang out with other species from time to time.

Only days after the announcement of quotas by the Faroese government, to add salt to the festering wound, on 29th July 2022, one hundred bottlenose dolphins were massacred. The official figures only claim 97, however they also claim them to be Atlantic white-sided dolphins when they very clearly were not. The slaughter occurred at the very same beach and was overseen by the very same sheriff, who gave the green light to murder 1,423 souls almost a year before. Local news reported, this was the first time, the *'new dolphin killing tool'* was used. The despicable sheriff was quoted as saying *'the killing went smoothly'* - *(Can someone please shoot this disgusting sheriff...!)* Somehow, the remainder of the world feels certain the dolphins did not feel the same way. It is beyond heart-breaking.

One of the overarching concerns surrounding the hunting of Atlantic white-sided dolphins is their conservation status and the fact that little is known about the species or the threats they face. It's unlikely they can withstand additional pressure from hunting. The same can be said for bottlenose dolphins. We know so little about the North East Atlantic dolphin population, but we do know, the Faroes are likely to bring about the extinction of these vulnerable populations.

Instead of listening to the science, both conservation and human-health-related, to their own citizens, industry, tourism and international political pressure, the powers that be within Faroese society have decided to allow the continued and expanded slaughter of innocent lives, by a small minority of islanders. It's time for the majority to stand up for what they believe in. The **WDC** are working to help the dolphins have their precious voices heard.

Original Report - *Nicola Hodgins*

Please, stand together and boycott this terrible island, no matter what it takes. If anyone has anything to add or can provide help or financial aid to stop these Faroes Island people from continuing on their blood lust campaign to destroy the innocent dolphins and whales of our world, then please contact the ***Whale and Dolphin Conservation (WDC)*** who are the leading global charity dedicated to the protection of whales and dolphins. They care deeply about whales and dolphins and they share this passion with their supporters. They have integrity, their work is backed by robust research, science and philosophy. These are the good guys out there saving innocent lives every day. Please support them…!

5.) Sharks

For 400 million years, sharks have roamed every ocean on earth. Few species have thrived on our planet for as long and fewer have been so misunderstood. These mysterious, magnificent predators are essential to the balance of marine ecosystems. Sharks have survived five mass extinctions, including the extinction that killed the dinosaurs…!

Today, there are approximately 470 known species of sharks living in our oceans. However, nearly one in four of these species are currently threatened with extinction due to human activities, like overfishing and shark finning. According to the *International Union for Conservation of Nature (IUCN)*, the list of endangered shark species is surprisingly long. Among the approximately 470 species of sharks, 2.4% are listed as Critically Endangered, 3.2% Endangered, 10.3% Vulnerable, and 14.4% Near Threatened.

Sadly, humans kill up to 100 million sharks per year. Worldwide, sharks are targets of vast overfishing to supply the enormous, repulsive demand for shark fin soup, a delicacy served at high-level social and diplomatic functions in Asia, particularly in Japan.

Sharks are actually more valuable to humans for non-consumptive reasons, like ecotourism, smart design and most importantly; management of the ocean's carbon cycle. This gives some hope for shark conservation efforts around the world.

Sharks boost local economies through ecotourism. Over the last several decades, public fascination with sharks has developed into a thriving ecotourism industry in places such as the Bahamas, South Africa and the Galápagos Islands. These activities, which support businesses like boat rental and diving companies, are said to provide 10,000 jobs in 29 countries.

Shark's streamlined anatomy has inspired smart design such as watercraft, cars and water turbines. Science has been practicing biomimicry, imitating nature's designs to solve human problems for many years.

The world's biggest shark, the whale shark, can grow as long as 40 feet. As filter-feeders, whale sharks swim with their mouths open to passively filter-feed on small fish, invertebrates and plankton. While whale sharks aren't as popularized in media as the jagged-toothed great whites, they do have a considerable impact on coastal economies around the world, attracting large amounts of dive tourism. In the United States, some buyers regard the whale shark and the basking shark as trophy species. They pay a staggering $10,000 to $20,000 for a single fin. We sadly have some seriously sick humans inhabiting our planet…!

The top shark hunting nations are: Indonesia, India, Spain, Taiwan, Argentina, Mexico, Pakistan, the United States, Japan, and Malaysia, with Thailand, France, Brazil, Sri Lanka, New Zealand, Portugal, Nigeria, Iran, the United Kingdom and South Korea, comprising the top twenty shark fishing nations. Japan alone has an annual average catch of almost 25,000 tonnes…!

Nearly every fin of a shark is targeted for harvest. The primary and secondary dorsal fins are removed from the top of the shark, plus its pectoral fins. In a single cutting motion, the pelvic fin, anal fin and bottom portion of its caudal fin, are removed. Because the rest of the shark has little value the finless and still-living shark is thrown back into the sea to free space aboard the vessel. Unable to swim effectively, they sink to the bottom of the ocean and die from lack of oxygen because they're not able to move to filter the water through their gills. Alternatively, they are eaten slowly by other smaller *nibbling* predators.

Shark finning at sea enables fishing vessels to increase profitability and increase the number of sharks harvested, as they only store and transport the fins, which are by far the most profitable part of the shark; whereas, the shark meat is bulky to transport. Many countries have banned this practice, requiring the whole shark to be brought back to port before removing the fins.

Shark finning has increased since 1997 largely due to

the increasing demand for fins for shark fin soup and traditional cures, particularly in China and the Asian territories. Thankfully, some shark fin soup substitutes have lately appeared on the market, which do not require any real shark fins.

The *International Union for Conservation of Nature's Shark Specialist Group,* claim shark finning is widespread, rapidly expanding and largely unregulated. The shark fin trade represents one of the most serious threats to shark populations worldwide. Shark fins are among the most expensive seafood products, commonly retailing at US$400 per kg and more...

Shark finning has caused catastrophic harm to the marine ecosystem. A variety of shark species are now seriously threatened, including the critically endangered Scalloped Hammerhead shark. Sharks have a K-selection life history, which means, they tend to grow slowly, reach maturity at a larger size and a later age and they have low reproductive rates. These traits make them especially vulnerable to overfishing methods, such as shark finning. Recent studies suggest, numbers of some shark species have dropped as much as 80% over the last fifty years, primarily due to shark finning and bycatch (the unintentional capture of species by other fisheries).

Sharks are apex predators. Their loss creates extensive implications for marine systems and processes, like coral reefs. *'Live Science'* said the following: 'The overfishing of sharks have serious effects for the entire marine food chain in some ecosystems. Removing sharks from a reef environment in the Caribbean had an effect on other species. Without sharks, carnivorous fish, which sharks usually fed on, thrived. The carnivorous fish, in turn, preyed on parrotfish who kept the corals clean. In time, the reefs changed from one dominated by coral to one overrun by algae.' - *Source Wikipedia*

Fins from the critically endangered sawfish (**Pristidae**) are also highly favoured in Asian markets. They are some of the most valuable. Sawfish are now protected under the highest protection level of the Convention on International Trade in Endangered Species. Sadly, their numbers continue to dwindle due to illegal poaching.

And we were given this world for free…! When will this despicable carnage stop…? When will mankind realise, we are killing our planet…sigh…

6.) Whales

Whales roam throughout all of the world's oceans, communicating via a series of complex and mysterious sounds. Their sheer size is amazing, the blue whale can reach lengths of more than 100 feet and weigh up to 200 tons, which equates to approximately 33 elephants…! These are seriously big guys, peacefully existing around our oceans.

Despite living in the water, whales breathe air. Like humans, they are warm-blooded mammals who nurse their young. A thick layer of fat called blubber, insulates them from cold ocean waters. Being warm-blooded they are sentient beings, they experience emotions. They know pain and fear, like all of us…

Some whales are named baleen whales, including blue, right, bowhead, sei and grey whales. This is because they have special bristle-like structures in their mouths (called baleen) that strain food from the water. Other whales, such as beluga or sperm whales, have teeth. Humpback whales make some of the longest migrations on earth. Scientists tracked one whale who travelled 11,770 miles over 265 days from its summer foraging area near the Antarctic Peninsula up to its winter breeding area off Colombia and back again to the Antarctic Peninsula.

Throughout the Southern Hemisphere, humpbacks make seasonal migrations between the tropics and polar waters, moving along the coasts through the waters of 28 countries and the open ocean, mostly lying beyond the jurisdiction of any nation. However, the growing dangers whales face worldwide along these epic journeys are signs of an ocean in peril and reveal how these waters actually connect us all.

Whales are essential to a healthy ocean and planet. Along their migrations, whales fertilize the marine ecosystems they move through and support the marine life inhabiting them. Their faecal plumes boost phytoplankton production, which captures about 40% of all carbon dioxide produced, generating over half of the atmosphere's oxygen. When they die, whales sink to the seabed, taking massive amounts of carbon out of the atmosphere for centuries. Altogether, one whale captures the same amount of carbon over its lifetime as thousands of trees. This means, by restoring whale populations, we can help restore ocean ecosystems and mitigate and build resilience to climate change. It's helping nature help itself, including all of us who depend on it.

Despite the vital role they play in the health of our planet and our own lives, whales constantly face a barrage of new and growing threats from humans. As many as 300,000 whales, including dolphins and porpoises are killed every year from entanglement in fishing gear. Ever-expanding shipping traffic, leads to more collisions between whales and ships. Ship traffic, also creates serious underwater noise disturbance for these gentle giants.

The countries where commercial whale hunting continues are - Japan, Norway and Iceland. Norway kills the most whales of the three countries. Please boycott these disgusting countries. Iceland announced in February 2022, it would stop its commercial whaling practices by 2024. We're watching…

Climate change is shifting whale prey populations, especially in the polar regions, making it harder for them to find food. Eight million tons of plastic are entering the sea every year. This is about one full garbage truck every minute. New research shows, whales near large cities ingest around three million microplastics per day. Is there anything humans do that is actually good for our planet..?

The crisis unfolding in our ocean is impacting the recovery and health of whale populations in different ways around the globe. While the moratorium on commercial whaling allowed some populations to recover from the brink of extinction, some have not. Six out of the thirteen great whale species are now classified as endangered or vulnerable. North Atlantic right whales are at their lowest point in about 20 years, numbering only 366 individuals, a decline of 30% over the past 10 years.

For the first time, *Protecting Blue Corridors*, a new report by *WWF* and *Oregon State University, University of California Santa Cruz, University of Southampton* and others, monitor the satellite tracks of over 1000 migratory whales worldwide. They identify where migratory routes and key habitat areas overlap with human activities like shipping, which helps to better protect and manage ocean habitats worldwide.

WWF are calling for collaboration among researchers, local communities, national and international policymakers, governments and industry to protect blue corridors by securing critical ocean habitats for whales.

The idea is to implement a comprehensive network of marine protected areas overlapping national and international waters by 2030. This will help protect and conserve whales and many other species, while strengthening the ocean's resilience to climate change. Their objective is to:

1. Work to achieve *'zero bycatch'* in fisheries in national and international waters
2. Eliminate and clean up *'ghost gear'*, abandoned, lost, or otherwise discarded fishing gear
3. Establish an ambitious UN global treaty to stop the leakage of plastics into our ocean by 2030 and move ships away from critical whale habitats where possible
4. Set ship slow-down rules and other measures to reduce underwater noise and risks of ship strikes
5. Invest in whales for a thriving ocean by integrating the vital ecological role of whales into global and national climate and biodiversity policies

Together, we can protect these ocean giants and make their epic journeys safer for years to come. *- Courtesy WWF*

7.) Rhinos

Rhinos once roamed throughout Europe, Asia and Africa. They were known to early Europeans who depicted them in cave paintings. Within historical times, they were still widespread across Africa's savannas and Asia's tropical forests. Today, very few rhinos survive outside protected areas. All five species are threatened, primarily from poaching and hunting.

By 1970, rhino numbers dropped to 70,000 and today, only around 27,000 rhinos remain in the wild. Very few rhinos survive outside national parks and reserves due to persistent poaching, hunting and habitat loss over many decades. Three species of rhino; Black, Javan and Sumatran, are critically endangered.

Rhinoceroses are universally recognized by their massive bodies, stumpy legs and either one or two dermal horns. In some species, the horns may be short or not obvious. They are renowned for having poor eyesight, but their senses of smell and hearing are well developed. The biggest of the five surviving species are Africa's white rhino and Asia's greater one-horned rhinos. These two species have thankfully seen their numbers increase in recent years due to successful conservation efforts. The white rhino is now classified as near threatened, while the greater one-horned rhino has moved from endangered to vulnerable.

However, they still remain at real risk from poaching, which has seen a dramatic increase since 2008. This poses a major threat to the survival of all rhino species, particularly Africa's endangered black rhino and Asia's critically endangered Javan and Sumatran rhinos. But there is hope. The white and greater one-horned rhinos were saved from extinction. Black rhino numbers have also increased, although they are still just a fraction of their number fifty years ago.

Although international trade in rhino horn has been banned under **CITES (Convention on International Trade in Endangered Species of Fauna and Flora)** since 1977, demand remains high, particularly in Vietnam (upper-middle class citizens) but the problem is essentially rife throughout the eastern countries like China, Korea, etc. Powdered horn is used in traditional Asian medicine as a supposed cure for a range of illnesses, from hangovers to fevers and even cancer. As well as its use in medicine, rhino horn is also bought and consumed purely as a symbol of wealth.

There has been a huge surge in poaching since 2008, particularly in South Africa, which has seen record numbers of rhinos poached in recent years. Poaching gangs (supported by wealthy criminal syndicates) use increasingly sophisticated methods to evade authorities, including helicopters and night vision equipment to track rhinos and they us veterinary drugs to knock them out. Governments and conservationists need to match this level of technology to tackle the problem.

Habitat loss also threatens rhinos, especially in southeast Asia and India, as human populations rise and forests are degraded or destroyed. Important core conservation areas are increasingly isolated by logging, agricultural expansion, human settlements, road projects and dam construction. Asian rhinos mainly survive in isolated areas, in small populations, which are at risk from inbreeding, natural disasters and disease.

WWF is helping to tackle the major threats by strengthening protected areas in Africa and Asia, preserving rhino habitat and helping to stamp out the illegal trade in rhino horn, expanding protected areas, creating new ones, connecting isolated rhino habitats and increasing security in the following areas: Promoting wildlife-based tourism that helps fund conservation efforts and gives local communities an income from living alongside wildlife; Working with communities living around protected areas to help them use their natural resources more sustainably; and supporting the translocation of rhinos to create new, secure populations.

How can you help...?

Don't buy rhino horn products. The illegal trade in rhino horn poses the greatest threat to rhinos today. Adopt a Sumatran rhino through *WWF-US*. Adopt a rhino through *WWF-UK*. Use and support sustainable wood, paper and palm oil.

By purchasing certified sustainable palm oil and FSC-certified forest products, retailers and manufacturers help protect Sumatran and Javan rhino habitat by limiting illegal logging and forest conversion.

Consumers can help by demanding certified products and donating to *WWF* to support their work in Africa and Asia. – *Courtesy of WWF*

8.) Lions – Canned Hunting

Canned hunting allows wealthy, bloodlust hunters from overseas to shoot easy prey in Africa, in the form of innocent lions. The lions are bred solely for the purpose of being shot in cold blood for maximum profit. With Canned Hunting, the typically captive-bred animals are kept in fenced areas with no chance of escape. The ill-fated animals are directly served up to the hunters and simply shot. Because these lions are bred on farms and reared by hand, they are not shy of humans. Occasionally, they are attracted with bait and sometimes they are even sedated, making it easier for the *'brave'* hunter to execute the defenceless animal.

Situated on lion farms in South Africa, young lion cubs are reared in small pens. The cubs are adorably cute, with soft grubby brown fur and adorable eyes that miss nothing. These cubs are not wild, they are tame, they accept humans because for a modest fee, tourists stop by to pet and hug the playful, juvenile cats, little realising, nearby there are larger pens holding as many as fifty fully-grown lions and even a couple of tigers.

Sadly, there are more than 160 such farms legally breeding big cats in South Africa. More lions are currently held in captivity (upwards of 5,000) compared to free lions existing in the country's vast Game Parks (about 2,000).

Animal Welfare groups conclude: breeders sell their stock, knowing full well, they will be shot by wealthy trophy-hunters from Europe and North America. The hunters usually take the lion's head for a trophy mount. The left-over carcass is in huge demand for traditional medicine in Asia. It's rather like shooting fish in a barrel. A fully-grown, captive-bred lion is taken from its pen to an enclosed area where it wanders listlessly for some hours before being shot dead by a man with a shotgun, hand-gun or even a crossbow, standing safely on the back of a truck. He pays anything from £5,000 to £25,000, and unbelievably, it's all completely legal in South Africa.

Game Ranches invite tourists to enjoy *'Canned Hunting'* of anything from humble blesbok and beautiful springbok (South Africa's national symbol), to lions and even crocodiles. Tourists go on a Game Drive on a specially designed off-road vehicle (Land Rover), through the vast estates. Herds of blue wildebeest, red hartebeest and eland run on sight of the truck, then stop and watch, warily. According to the guides, the animals seem to know when visitors are not carrying guns.

Most of the animals look well cared for but it's all a smoke screen. For the lioness, cubs are removed from their mother an hour after birth and bottle-fed by humans for the first eight weeks of their life. Animal Welfare experts say breeders remove the cubs from their mother so the lioness will quickly become fertile again. The disgusting breeders squeeze as many cubs from an adult mother as possible. They get approximately five litters every two years. For an animal that is usually weaned at six months, missing out on the crucial colostrum, or first milk, can cause ill-health.

Says **Pieter Kat, an evolutionary biologist** who has worked with wild lions in Kenya and Botswana. 'Lions and tigers in captivity may kill their young because they are under a lot of stress. But the main reason breeders separate the young from their mother is because they don't want them to be dependent on their mother. Separation brings the female back into a reproductive position much faster than if the cubs were around. It's a *'sick'* conveyor-belt production of animals.'

South Africa has a strong hunting tradition but few people express much enthusiasm for its debased canned form. It's still legal to bring a lion carcass back to Britain (or anywhere in Europe or North America) as a trophy. Much of the demand comes from overseas. Trophy-hunters are attracted by the guarantee of success and the price: a wild lion shot on a safari in Tanzania may cost £50,000, compared with a £5,000 captive-bred specimen in South Africa.

Five years ago, the South African government effectively banned Canned Hunting by requiring an animal to roam free for two years before it could be hunted, severely restricting breeders and hunters' profitability. But lion breeders challenged the policy in South Africa's courts and a high court judge eventually ruled, such restrictions were not rational. The number of trophy-hunted animals has since soared. In the five years to 2006, 1,830 lion trophies were exported from South Africa; in the five years to 2011, 4,062 were exported, a 122% increase with the vast majority being captive-bred animals.

Demand from the Far East is also driving profits for lion breeders. In 2001, two lions were exported as *'trophies'* to China, Laos and Vietnam; in 2011, 70 lion trophies were exported to those nations. While the trade in tiger parts is now illegal, demand for lion parts for traditional Asian medicine is soaring. In 2009, five lion skeletons were exported from South Africa to Laos; in 2011, it was 496. The legal export of lion bones and carcasses has also soared. 'It's definitely a rapidly growing source of revenue for these canned breeding facilities,' says ***Will Travers of the charity 'Born Free'.*** 'The increases and volumes are staggering…!'

Breeders argue it is better that hunters shoot a captive bred lion than further endanger the wild populations, but conservationists and animal welfare groups dispute this. Wild populations of lions have declined by 80% in 20 years, so the rise of lion farms and canned hunting has not protected wild lions. In fact, according to ***Fiona Miles, director of Lions Rock,*** a big cat sanctuary in South Africa run by the charity, ***'FOUR PAWS'***, says it is actually fuelling it. The lion farms' creation of a market for canned lion hunts puts a clear price-tag on the head of every wild lion. They create a financial incentive for local people, who collude with poachers or turn a blind eye to illegal lion kills.

Trophy-hunters who begin with a captive-bred lion may then graduate to the real, wild thing. 'It's factory-farming of lions, and it's shocking,' says Miles. She began working to protect lions after watching a seminal documentary about Canned Hunting. 'The lion, all around the world, is known as the iconic king of the jungle. This is how it's portrayed in advertising and written into story books. Now, people have reduced it to a commodity, something that can be traded, used and abused.'

An alternative use for the captive-bred lions is tourism. *'Lion Walks' with Martin Quinn*, a conservation educator and lion whisperer, involves strolling through the veld with three adolescent white lions, which have been bred and trained by Quinn. Armed only with sticks, Quinn controls them, while warning tourists, they are still wild animals. It's an unnerving experience, but Quinn hopes this venture will persuade breeders, a live lion is worth more than a dead one. He claims, since he began working with lions at the ranch where he works, the owners haven't sold any lions to be hunted. He hopes the ranch will eventually allow the offspring of its captive animals to grow up in the wild. Breeders sometimes claim their lions are for conservation programmes but examples of captive-bred lions becoming wild animals again are vanishingly rare; even the most respectable zoo has never established a successful programme for releasing captive-bred lions into the wild.

Lions Rock, is a former lion breeding farm transformed into a sanctuary for more than 80 abused big cats, since it was bought by **FOUR PAWS**. Some lions come from local breeding farms, but **FOUR PAWS** also rescue animals kept in appalling conditions in zoos in Romania, Jordan and the Congo. Unlike in the lion farms, the animals here are not allowed to breed. Instead they live within large enclosures in their natural prides, with family groups of up to ten lions.

Lions Rock can rehouse another 100 lions but does not have space for every captive-bred lion in South Africa. **FOUR PAWS** and other charities working in South Africa want a moratorium on lion breeding because they fear, if lion farms were abruptly outlawed, thousands of lions would be dumped or killed. After its high court defeat, there is little sign the South African government will take on the powerful lion breeders again any time soon, considering the Prime Minister himself owns Game Farms for hunting. Original article - *Patrick Barkham*

'If we can stop people supporting those industries in the first place and make them aware of what's actually going on and what the life of a captive-bred lion is actually like, I believe there will be an outcry,' says Miles.

Lion breeders are well aware of the huge international dollar rich market, frothing to shoot lions. These particular gun happy yanks are the most prime evil destroyers of the African large animal kingdom. They all know, you come to Africa to shoot a lion, a rhino or an elephant and have the animal's head-mounted against your wall back home to prove, 'This is what I shot, that's how hardcore, tough I am…!'. Despicable sicko's, every one of them…!

9.) Cross Border Animal Trafficking

Millions of live animals and reptiles are smuggled across borders, cooped up in tiny containers. Few make it. The revulsion stories are endless.

Wildlife trade is big business, with illegal wild plants, rare lumber and exotic animals sold around the globe. It's also a leading cause of the planet's accelerating biodiversity crisis and resultant ecosystem collapse. Wildlife trade means, poaching and selling dead or living plants and animals and the products derived from them. Some of this is legal. But much of it isn't. Indeed, the **U.S. State Department** estimates, wildlife trafficking is the third-largest type of illegal trade, after drugs and weapons, with the value of smuggled goods totalling around $10 billion a year and climbing.

Why do people covet these species…? Animals such as Asian otters, squirrel monkeys and African grey parrots may be wanted as pets. Plus, their meat may be in demand as a delicacy in many countries. In fact, the rarer an animal, the greater the people's desire is to consume it; hence the hunger for pangolin meat and shark fins. Animal skins and hides, such as zebra, buck, giraffes or crocodiles, are highly sought for rugs or as leather for handbags and shoes. Their body parts may also be coveted for use in traditional Asian medicines. In particular, pangolin scales, sun bear bile and tiger bones are in huge demand. Whereas, elephant ivory is still seen as a status symbol. Plants, including wood from trees that are already excessively logged, are in demand for furniture or ornamental or medicinal purposes.

We are currently experiencing an extinction crisis. Since 1970 the planet has lost 60 percent of its vertebrate wildlife populations. The world's foremost experts have warned of an impending annihilation of certain wildlife. It is now an emergency, threatening civilization.

The United Nations Intergovernmental Science-Policy Platform on Biodiversity and Ecosystem Services (IPBES) report, concluded, one million species face extinction due to human causes, many within mere decades. Globally, wildlife trade is the second-biggest threat to the vital biodiversity of our planet, following habitat loss. A recent study found, 958 species have been listed at risk by the *International Union for Conservation of Nature (IUCN).* They are nearing extinction because they are essentially being traded internationally.

And it's once again, all about human greed and profit.

This has devastating impacts not only on wildlife itself, but also on humans. In fact, many scientists assert, the destruction of nature is as dangerous to human life as climate change and will probably threaten human life sooner than global warming because it results in cascading effects, reducing overall ecosystem functioning.

Indeed, we depend on biodiversity, meaning a wide range of species existing together on the planet, for the healthy soil and crops that provide our food, the water we drink, the clean air we breathe and the stability of weather patterns. An estimated four billion people also rely on natural medicines for their health care, medicines whose ingredients could be destroyed by a loss of biodiversity.

Illegal wildlife trade (what many refer to as *'wildlife crime'*), is also used to finance conflict, which contributes to instability in countries. In Central African countries, such as the Democratic Republic of Congo, some armed groups raise funds by poaching and selling animals and boards.

Destroying wildlife also has a severe economic impact on nations around the world. For example, logging and other forms of deforestation in Kenya, threaten the country's ability to grow tea, a product that brings in millions of dollars as an export industry.

The golden triangle of Laos, Thailand and Myanmar is a global hub for illegal wildlife trade and trafficking.

China is the largest importer of illegal wildlife and animal products, driving demands for animals, in particular from countries like South and Southeast Asia; Southern Africa; Zimbabwe (the country with the biggest poaching problem); and Kenya. The numbers of invasive alien species per country have risen by some seventy percent since 1970. The most popular animals in demand are Pangolins; African Rhinos; African Elephants; Tigers, and Abalone - as follows:

Pangolins

An estimated one million pangolins have been poached in the last decade, making them the most trafficked mammals in the world. These shy creatures are poached in Asia and Africa for their scales and body parts; consumed for nourishment, a symbol of wealth and for traditional medicine.

African Rhinos

Black and White Rhinos are among Africa's most iconic mega-fauna, gentle grazers and browsers who once spanned the entire continent. After years of ruthless poaching by organised criminal syndicates for their keratin horn, both African species of rhino are now threatened with extinction in the wild. They are in desperate need of constant protection throughout Africa. Sadly, it's not only poaching but also big game hunting safaris that contribute to these lovable animals growing extinction.

African Elephants

African Elephants are arguably the most well-known species to be heavily impacted by illegal trade and wildlife crime, given that approximately 90% have been decimated within the last century. Global efforts to reverse this devastating onslaught on African Elephant populations have seen positive results but demand for ivory still exists and illegal traders remain as resourceful and ruthless as ever. By closing domestic ivory markets, which are contributing to poaching, significant steps have been taken towards ending a relentless and needless slaughter that has lasted for decades. There is still however so much still to be done as the poaching numbers steadily increase year on year.

Tigers

Tiger populations have been devastated by poaching, illegal trade, human-wildlife conflict and habitat loss. Once common across Asian range states, these magnificent big cats are now estimated to number approximately 3,800 in the wild. *TRAFFIC* monitors the illegal trade in tigers and found, an average of 110 individuals a year have entered the illegal trade chain in Asia over the last 16 years. As a result of such findings, Parties to *CITES* are now committed to phasing out tiger farming, which contributes to this trade and stimulates demand for their parts. In earlier years, wealthy tourists were encouraged to hunt Tigers from an Indian elephant's back. This was also a huge factor in the decline of Tiger numbers. Despite such positive moves, there's still a long way to go before wild tigers shed their endangered status.

Abalone

South African Abalone is the most heavily exported species in aquaculture, compared to anywhere in the world. A staggering 95% of South African Abalone exports go to Hong Kong, where it is it consumed as a delicacy or re-exported. Recent **TRAFFIC** surveys have revealed, approximately 65% of South Africa's abalone exports are harvested illegally. Organised criminal syndicates and even drug cartels are involved in the illegal trade, which is harming both local communities and abalone populations.

10.) Transportation of Animals by Ship

The transporting of live, innocent animals by ship from country to country is an incredibly cruel procedure. Unbelievably, it is condoned by mankind in our modern world and still happening every day. The journeys are long and torturous. Animals are literally shipped to an agonising death. The ships are vastly overcrowded. Animals fall sick, are injured and often die hideous deaths during transport. When they are loaded and unloaded in ports, many animals endure intolerable cruelty, especially in third world countries and even within the EU, particularly during loading. Every year, some 4.5 million cattle, pigs, sheep and goats are exported from the EU to third world countries. Mainly sheep and cattle are transported by sea to Libya, Jordan, Saudi Arabia, Lebanon, Egypt, Eritrea, Algeria, Georgia and other countries.

According to *'Behind the News'*, Africa is implicated in the supply of innocent donkeys for Chinese medicine. The report was released on World Donkey Day. The donkeys are shipped from various Africa ports to China. Upon docking in China, the innocent and bewildered donkeys are bludgeoned to death for their skins and to produce *'ejiao'*, a gelatine like substance used in Chinese traditional medicines. The report clearly shows, *'ejiao'* has no medicinal value. It is supposedly used to nourish the blood and enhance the immune system.

British charity, *'The Donkey Sanctuary'*, estimates, the demand from China for donkey's is as many as ten million donkeys per year, representing almost a quarter of the entire global donkey population. The *'ejiao'* market is expected to maintain a growth rate of fifteen percent annually. China's Ministry of Agriculture has included *'donkey'* as a target industry. Sadly, humans are an exceptionally destructive and cruel species.

Around 3 million sheep were exported by sea from

Romania in 2020. Germany exports tens of thousands of animals to third world countries by road and by sea every year, mainly cattle; it also exports calves to Spain to be fattened before some of them are further embarked on vessels for third world countries.

Many more EU countries export animals via sea in similar ways. Tragedies at sea keep repeating: thousands of sheep and hundreds of cattle had to wait and suffer on vessels when the Suez Canal was blocked in spring 2021; 2,600 cattle were killed after being stranded at sea for over three months on the vessels *Elbeik* and *Karim Allah* from December 2020 until March 2021; more than 14,000 sheep drowned when the *Queen Hind* capsized in November 2019, close to the port of Midia, Romania. And so, it continues unabated, year after year and all because of man's insatiable greed for consuming animal flesh and blood as food and other.

Animals transported from the EU to third countries are often embarked on ships, which don't even meet the minimum legal requirements for animal welfare. Most livestock vessels are old, converted cargo vessels. Over half of them pose a high risk to maritime safety. The animals needlessly suffer, kept in dark, hot basements with little food or water for the long, buffeting journey. The level of animal suffering and mental terror experienced on these arduous journeys, is unthinkable.

Numerous investigations in EU and third-country ports

reveal the same thing: animal cruelty is common when handling animals for transportation. Nobody knows how many animals are injured or die during transports to third countries or in the first few days after arriving at the destination. Once the animals have crossed the EU border, no one is responsible for reporting their health status or mortality.

FOUR PAWS has called for a ban on all live animal transports to third countries by sea and by land. If at all, only carcasses and/or genetic material should be exported. The European Parliament has established a Committee of Inquiry on live animal transports to investigate violations and shortcomings of the EU Regulation 1/2005, which will also inform the revision of the Regulation.

To-date, it's still business as usual, the innocent animal suffering continues daily. How terribly sad…sigh…

Original Article - *FOUR PAWS*

11.) The Dog Meat Trade...

It's really difficult to try and understand why some humans would even consider consuming man's best friend…? Dogs are part of the family; they have been for centuries. They are highly intelligent, sentient beings, capable of expressing emotions, almost on a par with humans. Surely, you cannot eat your best friend…? Sadly, mankind eats dogs and cats throughout Asia and are still doing so every day. This is beyond revulsion and has to stop...!

This horrific and barbaric animal abuse is practiced in China, South Korea, the Philippines, Thailand, Laos, Vietnam, Cambodia, Indonesia, Nagaland in northern India and some other eastern countries. Dogs are also known to be eaten in certain African countries such as Ghana, Cameroon, DRC and Nigeria. There are even reports, dogs are killed for personal consumption by some farmers in remote parts of Switzerland. However, nothing compares to the sheer scale of the despicable trade of innocent dogs across Asia.

The incredible injustice of Dog Meat Farming is where innocent, harmless dogs are farmed for their meat. The industry is completely under-regulated compared to other stock animals. These intelligent, sensitive animals are subjected to hell while they wait to be served up as food on a plate for ignorant, despicable humans.

An estimated 30 million dogs are killed for human consumption each year across Asia in a ruthless trade, involving terrible cruelty to animals and often, with criminal activity involved. Between ten and twenty million dogs alone are slaughtered in China; at least two million in South Korea and a million or so in Indonesia. Around five million in Vietnam, of which about 80,000 are imported from Thailand, Laos and Cambodia. Absolute figures are impossible to obtain because the dog meat trade is entirely unregulated and mostly, illegal.

In South Korea, dogs are intensively farmed for the meat trade in appallingly deprived conditions. The dogs are born and reared on specific dog meat farms in an endless cycle of breeding under the most horrendous and brutally cruel conditions.

The trade is well-organized, with high numbers of dogs stolen or taken from streets, transported over long distances and then viciously murdered. In the majority of Asian countries, the dogs killed are either family pets stolen from homes and gardens, roaming *'community'* dogs or strays snatched from streets. Dog and cat thieves use a variety of methods, including poison. They then sell the animals to traders and restaurant owners. It's quite common to find dogs on trucks headed to slaughterhouses still wearing their collars.

Severe animal suffering is endemic to the dog meat trade. The animals are crammed by the hundreds onto the backs of trucks, packed so tightly in cages, they are unable to move. These petrified dogs are then driven for days or even weeks. Mostly sick and badly mauled, many of the desolate animals die from suffocation, dehydration or heatstroke, long before they even reach their destination. In Vietnam, it is not uncommon for dogs to be violently force-fed with a tube down the throat in order to boost their weight before sending them to slaughter.

Dogs on South Korean meat farms are kept locked in small, barren metal cages, left exposed to the elements and given just enough food and water to keep them alive. *HSI* has uncovered appalling conditions where disease and mental distress are rampant, with many dogs showing obvious signs of sickness, depression, severe malnutrition and abnormal behaviour.

All of these dogs will eventually end up at a slaughterhouse, market or a restaurant. The method by which they are killed varies: in South Korea, the most common method for slaughtering a dog is by electrocution but hanging and beating are also used. In China and Vietnam, dogs are usually beaten to death with a metal pipe and then bled out from a cut to the throat or groin, but they can also be thrown, still conscious, into large drums of boiling water, for easier removal of the dog's coat. In some cases, the treatment of the animal prior to slaughter is deliberately cruel because of the misguided belief that torturing a dog prior to death results in better-tasting, adrenaline-rich meat.

A lot of people in China do not eat dog meat. A 2016 opinion polls shows 69.5 percent have never tried it. It is not part of mainstream Chinese culinary culture. There is a growing animal protection movement in the country that roundly opposes the dog meat trade. There are frequent and documented violent clashes between dog thieves and angry dog owners. In 2015, nearly 9 million Chinese citizens signed petitions in support of a legislative proposal to ban the slaughter of dogs and cats. More than

100,000 people attended a massive rally in Dalian city.

A 2014 poll taken in South Korea revealed, while just over half of those questioned, eat dog meat, the vast majority only consume occasionally. Dog meat is mostly consumed by older generations and for perceived health benefits, particularly during the *'Boknal'* days of summer. Younger South Koreans are far more likely to shun consuming dogs and cats. Polls show, 60.5 percent of under-30-year-olds have never eaten dog meat. Despite a declining participation in dog meat consumption, societal acceptance of a perceived right to eat whatever, remains relatively strong.

Consuming dog meat poses a significant threat to health, i.e. outbreaks of cholera, rabies and the deadly Trichinellosis, also called Trichinosis (a disease one gets from digesting meat from animals infected with the microscopic parasite Trichinella).

The **World Health Organisation** estimates, eating dog meat increases the risk of contracting cholera 20-fold; a number of recent large-scale outbreaks in Vietnam were directly linked to consuming dogs and cats. Rabies, which kills around 39,000 people across Asia annually, has been found in dogs traded for human consumption in China, Vietnam and Indonesia. Original Article - **Humane Society Int.**

If you're from East Asia and you're reading this, please do everything in your power to prevent this terrible carnage from continuing. Create petitions, rally support and raise awareness at government level because this shocking abuse on innocent animals has to stop. It's not only an embarrassment to your country but also to yourself because you live there…take action urgently please…!

12.) Seal Clubbing…

Each spring, the Canadian government authorizes fishermen to club or shoot to death hundreds of thousands of baby seals for their fur, according to the Humane Society of the United States. The vast majority of harp seals murdered are between only one and three months old (so sick…!). Humane reforms have had little effect on the resolve of activists to ban commercial sealing outright. Proposals for a more regulated hunt were notably rejected with the European Union's 2009 blanket ban on seal products.

Most of Canada's seal hunters are Inuk. Exact numbers of seals hunted are difficult to come by. The *Nunavut territorial government* estimates, its hunters take 35,000 seals per year. In 2016, the Atlantic hunt took about 70,000 harp and grey seals. In 2006 the numbers grew to an incredible 355,000 which is insane.

Canada really, really likes hunting seals. While it's possible to replace sealing revenue with a negligible outlay of the federal budget, defenders aren't standing up for the economics of seal hunting, claiming it's more a way of life. In a Canada where Indigenous communities, suffered greatly by losing touch with traditional ways of making a living, the Inuit communities are determined to hang on to one of their oldest links to the land. The same is true in Newfoundland and Labrador, where sealers often come from communities decimated by fishing closures.

It's why, in Ottawa, seal hunting is one of the few issues, which virtually every politician safely agrees on. Seal flesh is served in the Parliament Hill cafeteria. At least one governor general has eaten raw seal heart. When parliament discussed the creation of a National Seal Products Day last April, virtually the entire chamber agreed, regardless of region or party.

A by-product of the seal hunt is, thousands of pounds of seal meat, seal bones and seal organs end up being tossed into the ocean. Fact is, Newfoundlanders do eat seals; seal flipper pie is a local favourite. But there's simply no market to absorb the meat from 70,000 seals per year. Waste not want not – **Wake up Canada...!**

The big question - is seal clubbing cruel...? You decide. Clubs and hakapiks are the killing implement of choice. Guns are widely used for a preferred head shot but from a rocking boat it's not easy. Clubs are therefore used to bludgeon the innocent, wounded seals to death. Each of these killing methods is demonstrably, blood thirstily and satanically cruel, no matter how you judge it.

Sadly, both in the Arctic and the Atlantic there are also *'struck and lost'* seals, i.e., seals that are killed but sink to the bottom before they can be collected. One 2000 study from the ***Department of Fisheries and Oceans*** found, between two and ten per cent of young seals were killed without being collected. The rates were markedly higher when it came to older seals who had been shot in open water. Amongst seals one year or older, up to 50 per cent sink after being shot. They are never claimed. They are murdered in cold blood for nothing. Can the killers really be that immune to innocent death by their own cruel hands…?

The United States, which had been heavily involved in the sealing industry, now maintains a complete ban on the commercial hunting of marine mammals, with the exception of indigenous peoples who are allowed to hunt a small number of seals each year. Their sister country Canada, should ideally take a leaf from their good book…!

Seal Clubbing in Namibia

Release of the footage of a condemning video that went viral of a seal hunt, taken by conservation group ***'Earthrace Conservation'***, coincides with the start of this year's seal cull, which is expected to kill between 80/90,000 seal pups and around 6,000 bulls. Campaigners say the seals are murdered in order to sell their fat and fur, while the government has previously stated, they are killed to protect dwindling fish stocks, which they estimate at around 700,000 metric tons of fish lost annually to seals. The conservation group called on the Namibian government to stop the cull, saying, a ban in neighbouring South Africa in 1990 had no economic impact on the fishery.

The actual process is barbaric and terribly cruel. Terrified, innocent pups are rounded up, separated from their mothers and violently bludgeoned to death. An additional 6,000 bull seals are killed for their genitalia, which are thought to be an aphrodisiac in some cultures and therefore exported to Asia.

At 6:00am, the clubbing begins. At around 9:00am each morning, bulldozers clean up and restore the beach before the tourists arrive to view the colony, because all of this happens in a designated Seal Reserve, a Reserve that has ideally been created to supposedly *'protect'* the seals and offer visitors a chance to view them in their natural habitat. A despicable tourist *'catch'* of note, with a hideous, unseen bloodbath of innocent lives – how disgusting. **_Shame on you Namibia...!_**

Sadly, Namibia is the only country in the Cape fur seal's range in which commercial hunting is permitted. Sealing occurs on two mainland colonies, Cape Cross and Wolf/Atlas Bay. Commercial hunters are thought to hire around 160 part-time workers to kill the pups, which are between the ages of 7 and 11 months, using spiked wooden clubs.

Two foreign journalists filming the Namibian seal cull in 2009 were arrested on the grounds they had entered a protected marine area without a permit. One of them, was severely beaten by the seal hunters. The Namibian government declined to comment. Namibia and Canada are the only two countries in the world, who allow major seal culls. – Original Article - *John Vidal*

13.) Laboratory Testing on Animals

Imagine a syringe being forced down your throat to inject a chemical into your stomach or being restrained and forced to breathe sickening vapours for hours. This is the cruel reality of animal testing for millions of mice, rabbits, dogs and other animals, worldwide. Animal testing is legally required for many of the products we use every day. From fragrances to painkillers to the fabric dyes in clothing, every new chemical has at one time been force-fed to animals.

The term *'Animal Testing'* refers to procedures performed on living animals for purposes of research into basic biology and diseases, assessing the effectiveness of new medicinal products and testing the human health and/or environmental safety of consumer and industry products such as cosmetics, household cleaners, food additives, pharmaceuticals and industrial/agricultural chemicals.

All procedures, even those classified as mild, have the potential to cause the animals physical as well as psychological distress and suffering. Often the procedures can cause a great deal of suffering. Most animals are killed at the end of an experiment. Some are even re-used in subsequent experiments. This is a selection of common animal procedures:

1. Forced chemical exposure in toxicity testing, which can include oral force-feeding, forced inhalation, skin or injection into the abdomen, muscle, etc.
2. Exposure to drugs, chemicals or infectious disease at levels that cause illness, pain, distress and death
3. Genetic manipulation, e.g., addition or *'knocking out'* of one or more genes
4. Prolonged periods of physical restraint
5. Food and water deprivation
6. Surgical procedures followed by recovery
7. Infliction of wounds, burns and other injuries to study healing
8. Infliction of pain to study their physiology
9. Behavioural experiments designed to cause distress, e.g., electric shock or forced swimming
10. Other manipulations to create *'animal models'* of human diseases ranging from cancer to stroke to depression
11. Killing by carbon dioxide asphyxiation, neck-breaking, decapitation or other means

Many different species of animals are used around the world. The most common include mice, fish, rats, rabbits, guinea pigs, hamsters, farm animals, birds, cats, dogs, mini-pigs and primates (monkeys and in some countries, chimpanzees). It's estimated, more than 115 million animals worldwide are used in laboratory experiments every year. However, because only a small proportion of countries collect and publish data concerning animal use for testing and research, the precise number is unknown. For example, in the United States, up to 90 percent of the animals used in laboratories (purpose-bred rats, mice, birds, fish, amphibians, reptiles and invertebrates) are excluded from the official statistics, meaning, figures published by the U.S. Department of Agriculture are no doubt a substantial underestimate.

Within the European Union, more than 12 million animals are used each year, with France, Germany and the United Kingdom being the top three countries. British statistics reflect the use of more than three million animals each year. This number doesn't include animals bred for research but rather killed as surplus, without being used for specific experimental procedures. Although these animals still endure the stresses, pain and deprivation of life in a sterile laboratory environment, their lives are not recorded in official statistics.

For nearly a century, drug and chemical safety assessments have been based on laboratory testing, involving rodents, rabbits, dogs and other animals. Aside from the ethical issues they pose, i.e. inflicting both physical pain as well as psychological distress and suffering on large numbers of sentient creatures, animal tests are time and resource intensive. They are restrictive in the number of substances, which can be tested and they actually provide little understanding of how chemicals behave in the body. In many cases they do not correctly predict real-world human reactions. Similarly, health scientists are increasingly questioning the relevance of research aimed at *'modelling'* human diseases in the laboratory by artificially creating symptoms in other animal species.

Trying to mirror human diseases or toxicity by artificially creating symptoms in mice, dogs or monkeys has major scientific limitations, which cannot be overcome. Very often the symptoms and responses to potential treatments seen in other species are dissimilar to those of human patients. As a consequence, nine out of every ten candidate medicines that appear safe and effective in animal studies, fail when given to humans. Drug failures and research that never delivers because of irrelevant animal models, not only delay medical progress, they also waste resources and risk the health and safety of volunteers in clinical trials.

If a lack of human relevance is the fatal flaw of *'animal models'* then a switch to human-relevant research tools is the logical solution. The ***National Research Council*** in the United States, expressed its vision of a not-so-distant future in which virtually all routine toxicity testing would be conducted in human cells or cell lines. Science leaders around the world have echoed this view. The sequencing of the human genome and birth of functional genomics, the explosive growth of computer power and computational biology and high-speed robot automation of cell-based (in vitro) screening systems, to name a few, has sparked a quiet revolution in biology. Together, these innovations have produced new tools and ways of thinking, which help uncover exactly how chemicals and drugs disrupt normal processes in the human body at the level of cells and molecules. Scientists use computers to interpret and integrate this information with data from human and population-level studies. The resulting predictions regarding human safety and risk are potentially more relevant to people in the real world than animal tests.

The wider field of human health research could benefit from a similar shift in paradigm. Many disease areas have seen little or no progress despite decades of animal research. Some 300 million people currently suffer from asthma, yet only two types of treatment have become available in the last 50 years. More than a thousand potential drugs for stroke have been tested in animals but only one of these has proved effective in patients. And it's the same story with many other major human illnesses. A large-scale re-investment in human-based (not mouse or dog or monkey) research, aimed at understanding how disruptions of normal human biological functions at the levels of genes, proteins and cell and tissue interactions, lead to illness in our species, will advance the effective treatment or prevention of many key health-related societal challenges of our time.

Despite this growing evidence that it is time for a change, effecting change within a scientific community, which has relied for decades on animal models as the default method for testing and research, will take time and perseverance. Old habits die hard. Globally there is still a lack of knowledge and expertise in cutting-edge non-animal techniques. It's often argued, because animal experiments have been used for centuries and medical progress has been made in that time, animal experiments must be necessary. This is obviously missing the point. History is full of examples of flawed or basic practices and ideas that were once considered state-of-the-art, only to be superseded years later by something far more sophisticated and successful.

In the early 1900's, the Wright brothers' invention of the airplane was truly innovative for its time but more than a century later, technology advanced at such a rate, when compared to the modern jumbo jet, those early flying machines seem quaint and even absurd. Those early ideas are part of aviation history. However, no-one would seriously argue, they represent the cutting-edge of design or human achievement. So, it is with laboratory research.

Animal experiments are part of medical history but history is where they belong. Compared to today's potential to understand the basis of human disease at cellular and molecular levels, experimenting on live animals seems positively primitive. If we want better quality medical research, safer more effective pharmaceuticals and cures to human diseases, we need to turn the page in the history books and embrace the new chapter - 21st century science has arrived...!

Independent scientific reviews clearly demonstrate, research using animals, correlates very poorly to real human patients. In fact, the data show, animal studies fail to predict real human outcomes in 50 to 99.7 percent of cases. This is mainly because other species seldom naturally suffer from the same diseases as found in humans. Animal experiments rely on often uniquely human conditions being artificially induced in non-human species. While on a superficial level they may share similar symptoms, fundamental differences in genetics, physiology and biochemistry can result in wildly different reactions to both the illness and potential treatments.

For some areas of disease research, overreliance on animal models may well have delayed medical progress rather than advanced it. By contrast, many non-animal replacement methods such as cell-based studies, silicon chip biosensors and computational systems biology models, provide faster and more human-relevant answers to medical and chemical safety questions, which animal experiments cannot match.

The claim that animal experimentation is essential to medical development is not supported by proper, scientific evidence but by opinion and anecdote. Systematic reviews of its effectiveness don't support the claims made on its behalf.

Note the following very sad and unnecessary stats:

1. 10,000 Animals are killed for every new pesticide chemical tested
2. 32 Beagles are used in government-required tests for **EACH** new drug or agrochemical
3. Different animal species or routes of administration (oral force-feeding, forced inhalation or skin penetration); no pain relief is provided
4. There's no humane way to poison animals with chemicals or to infect them with deadly diseases like rabies to test the effectiveness of a vaccine; however, there are modern non-animal alternatives that work just as well, or better.

The *Humane Society International (HSI)* works through intergovernmental bodies such as the *OECD* to accelerate global adoption of modern non-animal testing methods. Via their network of country offices, they conduct the new approaches through national regulations. *(HSI)* have been instrumental in securing mandatory alternative requirements in Brazil and South Korea, whereby it is illegal for a company to conduct animal experimentation if a non-animal approach is available. They also help pass bans on cosmetic animal testing around the world through their *'Be Cruelty Free'* campaign. *HSI* are working around the globe in cooperation with companies and government authorities to replace cruel and obsolete animal-poisoning tests with modern alternatives, which better protect human and environmental safety. *Original Article - **Humane Society Int.***

What Can You Do...?

1. Never buy products that have been tested on animals. Look for the *'bunny'* symbol on the packaging

2. Support organizations like **NRDC; (HSI); FOUR PAWS; WDC; WWF; IUCN**; including all the other incredible groups who are constantly fighting to save animals

3. Contact your representatives in Congress, let them know you are concerned about Animal Laboratory Testing; Wildlife & Marine extinction; The Dog Meat Trade; Transportation of Animals by Ship; Cross Border Animal Trafficking; etc.

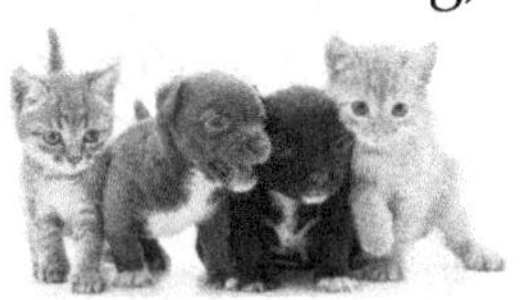

Make a concerted effort to boycott any company using animals to test their products. There are many companies who specialise in producing products completely free of animal testing. As consumers, the power is with us. Only support these *'animal free'* companies please…

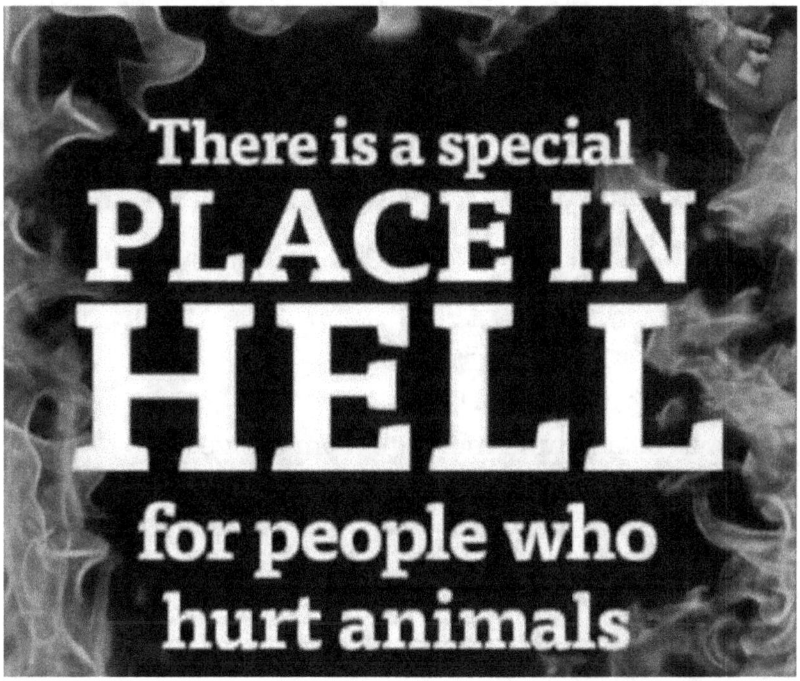

Traditional animal testing is expensive, time-consuming, uses a lot of animals and from a scientific perspective the results do not translate to humans - Dr Christopher Austin

The Dog Poem...

There were 1600 dogs
Living in a pen with hogs
Waiting for the butcher's knife
To bring an end to their life

Oh, how they screamed
When they saw the human steel
The beginning of the end
The human would them send

Maybe better than being starved
Stuck in a cage not very large
Desperate for some love
Or maybe a simple message from above

How does a human stoop so low…?
Animals have feelings don't you know
They are no better, no worse
Than any of us in which they trust

It's time for humans to let go
Live in harmony, go with the flow
Share our planet with deep respect
Equality and dignity, we'll accept

Robin Morris

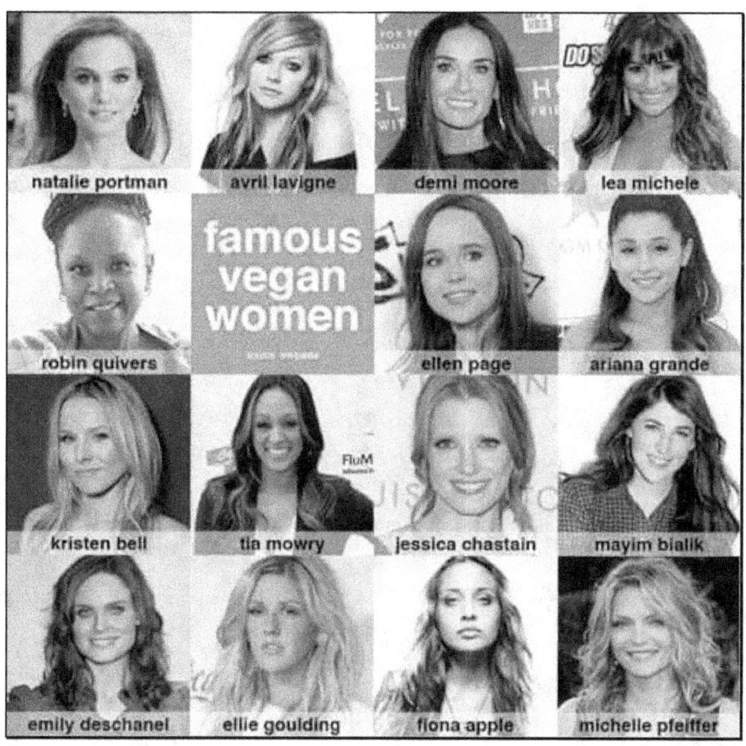

Vegan Quotes & Vegan Celebrities

There are famous actors/actresses, musicians, scientists, sportsmen/women and others, worldwide who proudly endorse a life of absolute veganism. For some, it's for health reasons, for others it's more about saving the animal kingdom and enforcing animal rights. Whatever their reasons, most of these global celebrities have collectively made a stand, using their fame and recognition, to support the current plight of the animal kingdom and stop the horrendous abuse and mismanagement of not only what is left of the world's marine and wildlife (currently in dire straits) but also domestic animals, which many of the world's eight billion population, consume daily. If you care to Google, *'Vegan Celebrities'*, you'll observe a long list of famous people supporting the animal cause. Listed below are some of the more popular quotes and appellations...

Quotes...

'I do it because I love animals and I saw the reality. And I just couldn't ignore it anymore. I'm healthier for it, I'm happier for it. I can't imagine, if you're putting something in your body that is filled with fear or anxiety or pain, that it isn't somehow going to be inside of you' - *Ellen DeGeneres*

'Violence begins with the fork' - *Mahatma Gandhi*

If you don't like pictures of animal cruelty being posted on social media, you need to help stop the cruelty, not the pictures. You should be bothered it's happening, not that you saw it' - *Marie Sarantakis*

'There is no fundamental difference between humans and animals in their ability to feel pleasure and pain, happiness, and misery' - *Charles Darwin*

'People eat meat and think they will become as strong as an ox, forgetting the ox eats grass' - *Pino Caruso*

'Poor animals, how jealously they guard their bodies, for to us its merely an evening's meal, but to them, it is life itself'
— *T Casey Brennan*

'Animal factories are one more sign of the extent to which our technological capacities have advanced faster than our ethics' - *Peter Singer*

'If slaughterhouses had glass walls, the entire world would be vegetarian' - *Linda McCartney*

'Could you look an animal in the eyes and say to it, 'My appetite is more important than your suffering' - *Moby*

'To kill an animal in order to satisfy your nutritional desires and not your nutritional needs, that to me is completely unacceptable' - *David Benatar*

'It takes nothing away from a human to be kind to an animal' - *Joaquin Phoenix*

'It's pretty amazing to wake up every morning, knowing every decision I make will cause as little animal harm as possible. It's a pretty fantastic way to live' - *Colleen Patrick-Goudreau*

'My body will not be a tomb for other creatures' - *Leonardo Da Vinci*

'Every living creature has the right to live ethically' - *D.V.*

'There are no negatives to eating vegan. I feel nothing but positive, mentally and physically. I love it. I feel like it also has a kind of a domino effect on the rest of my life' *Liam Hemsworth*

'Animals are my friends and I don't eat my friends...!' *George Bernard Shaw*

'The soul is the same in all living creatures, even though
the body of each is different' – *Hippocrates*

'I am a firm believer in eating a full plant-based, whole food
diet that can expand your life length and make you an all-
around happier person' - *Ariana Grande*

'It is my view, the vegetarian manner of living, by its
purely physical effect on the human temperament, would
most beneficially influence the whole of mankind'
Albert Einstein

'It is more important to prevent animal suffering, rather than
sit to contemplate the evils of the universe praying in the
company of priests' – *Buddha*

'A man of my spiritual intensity does not eat corpses'
George Bernard Shaw

'I don't see why someone should lose their life just so
you can have a snack' – *D.V.*

'If you knew how meat was raised, you wouldn't eat it'
Justin Timberlake

The day I stopped eating dairy, my sinuses and asthma also
stopped' – *E C Clapton*

'Veganism is not about giving anything up or losing
anything; it's about gaining the peace within that comes
from embracing nonviolence and refusing to participate in
the exploitation of the vulnerable' - *Gary L. Francione*

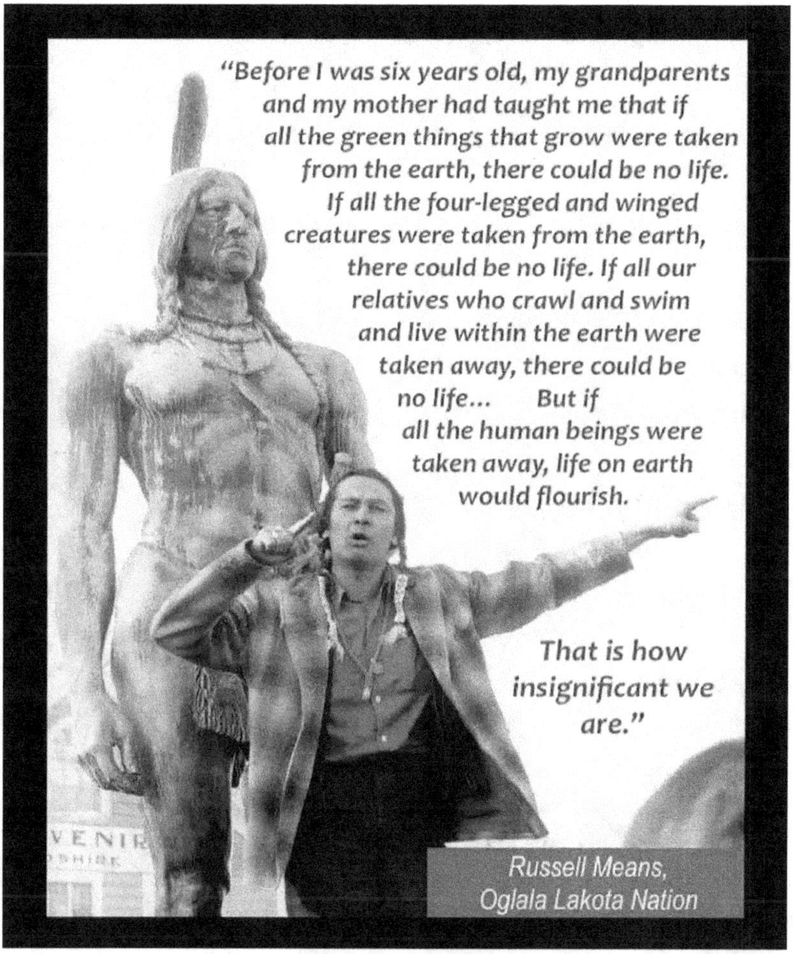

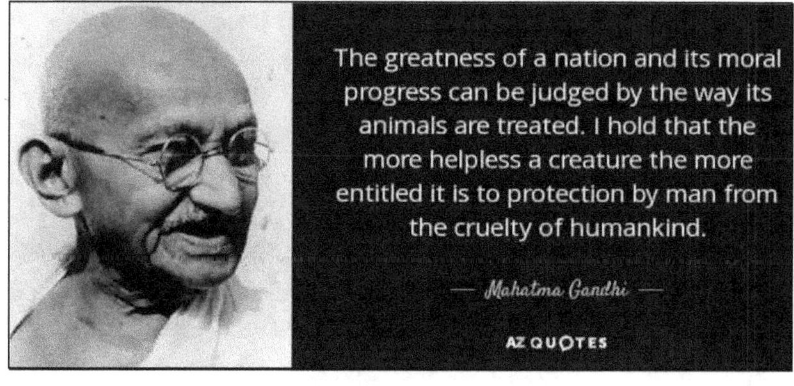

"Before I was six years old, my grandparents and my mother had taught me that if all the green things that grow were taken from the earth, there could be no life. If all the four-legged and winged creatures were taken from the earth, there could be no life. If all our relatives who crawl and swim and live within the earth were taken away, there could be no life... But if all the human beings were taken away, life on earth would flourish.

That is how insignificant we are."

Russell Means,
Oglala Lakota Nation

The greatness of a nation and its moral progress can be judged by the way its animals are treated. I hold that the more helpless a creature the more entitled it is to protection by man from the cruelty of humankind.

— Mahatma Gandhi —

AZ QUOTES

Celebrities - Vegan & Vegetarian

Arnold Schwarzenegger	Angelina Jolie
Keanu Reeves	Robert Downey Junior
Thandiwe Newton	Bill Gates
Liam Hemsworth	George W Bush
James Cameron	Beyonce'
Brad Pitt	Michelle Marie Pfeiffer
Jared Leto	Albert Einstein
Justin Timberlake	Steve Martin
Woody Harrelson	U2 Bono
Samuel L Jackson	Mike Tyson
Joaquin Phoenix	Bryan Adams
Russell Brand	Richard Branson
Miley Cyrus	Peter Dinklage
Forest Whitaker	Ricky Gervais

Anthony Kiedis

Alanis Morissette

River Phoenix

Alicia Silverstone

Jennifer Lopez

Alan Cummings

Colin Kaepernick

Leona Lewis

Mick Jagger

Sia

Larry Hagman

Tia Blanco

Scott Jurek

David Haye

Jay-Z

Eric Roberts

Billie Eilish

Morrissey

Lewis Hamilton

Brian May

James Cromwell

Meghan Markle

Roger Waters

Brooke Shields

Ariana Grande

Patrik Baboumian

Nate Diaz

Morgan Mitchell

The Bare Facts…

The following charts represent an easy guide to keep you updated with mineral and vitamin choices. You can copy and paste these charts into *'Word'*, enlarge them and print them out. Keep them in your cooking scrapbook or up on your kitchen wall for easy reference. The full colour version of this book is also available, which makes all the charts a lot easier to read…enjoy…!

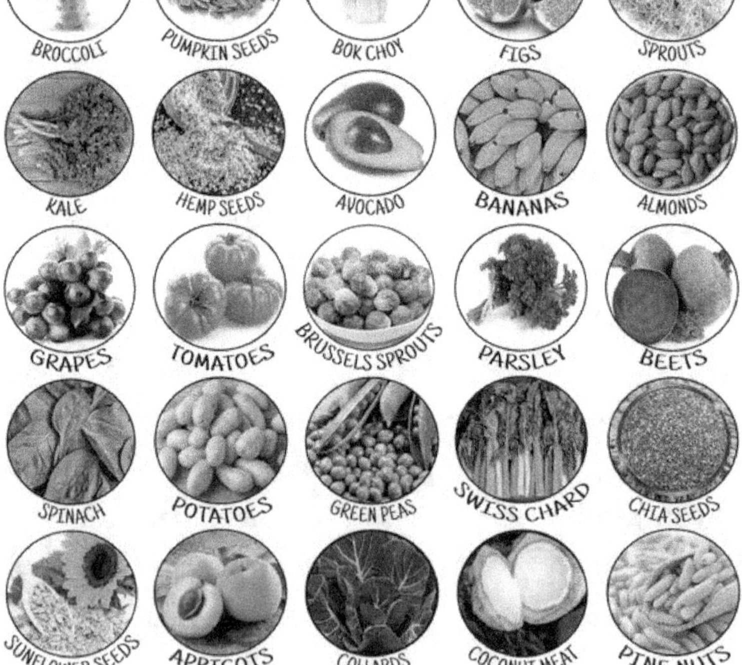

CALCIUM in PLANT FOODS

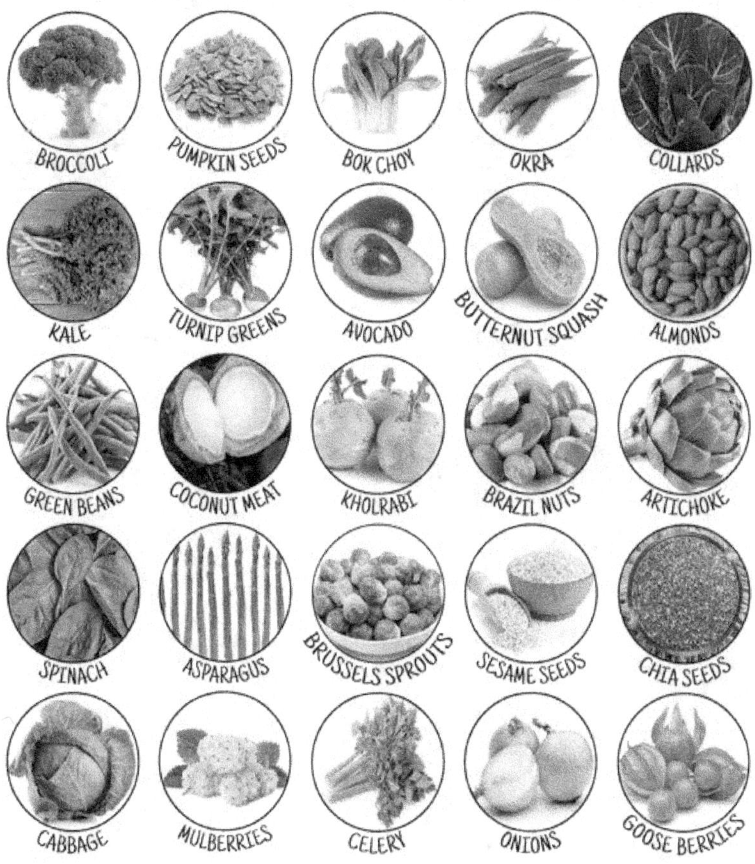

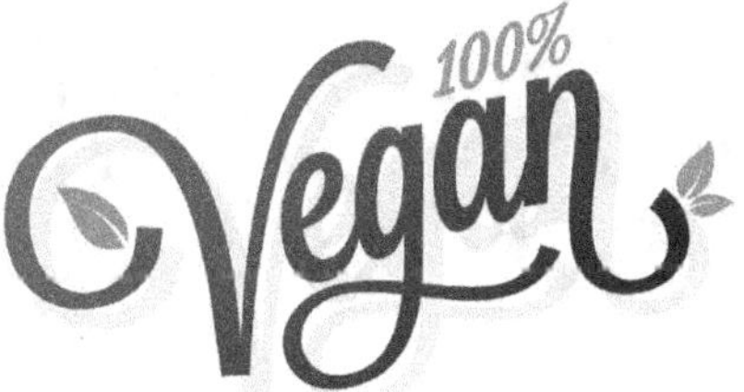

Fuel For MUSCLE GAINS

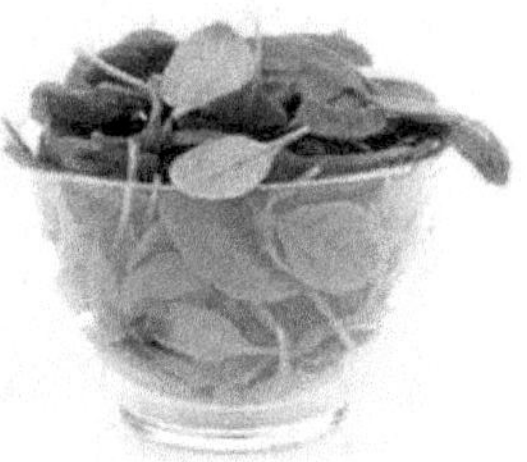

Spinach

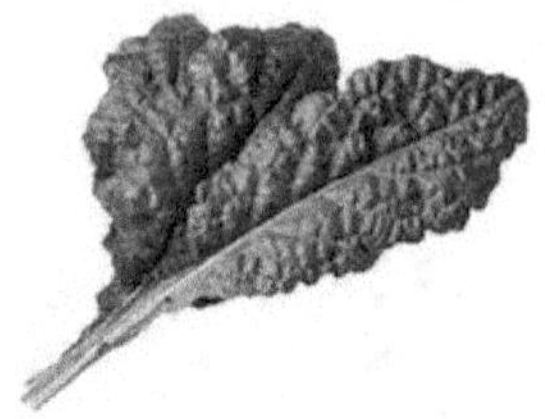

Kale

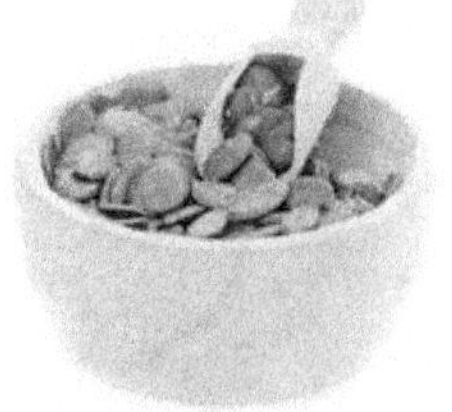

Pumpkin Seeds

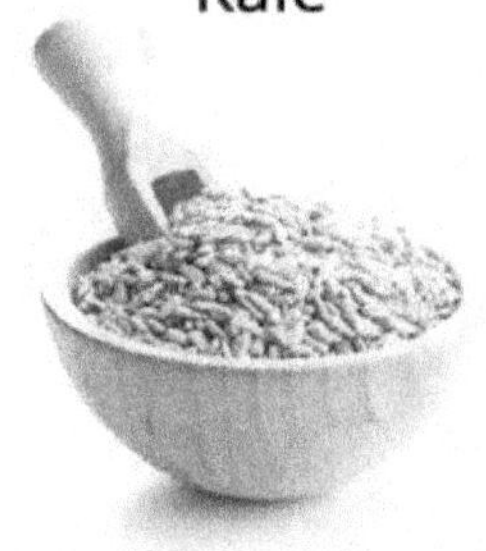

Sunflower Seeds

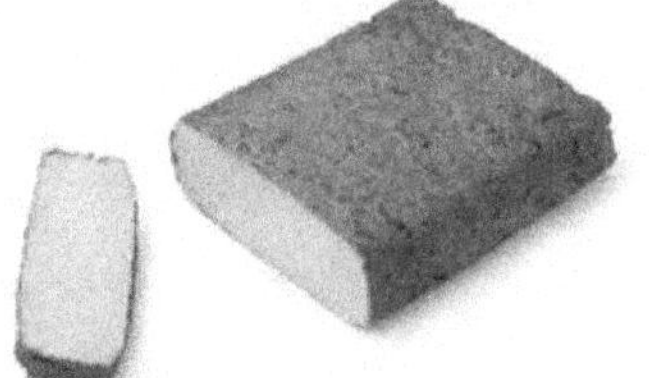

Tofu

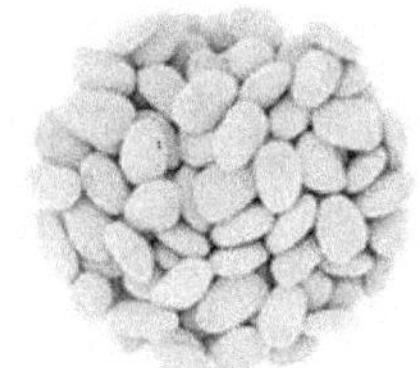

White Beans

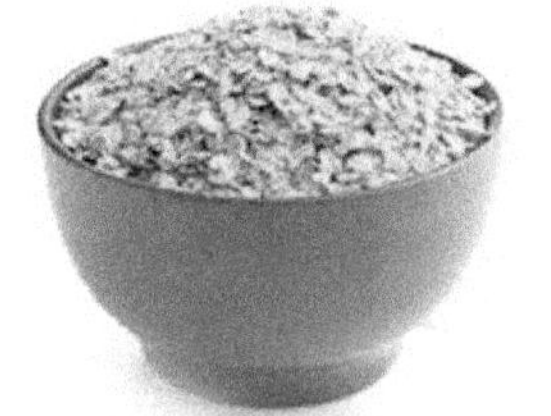

Oats

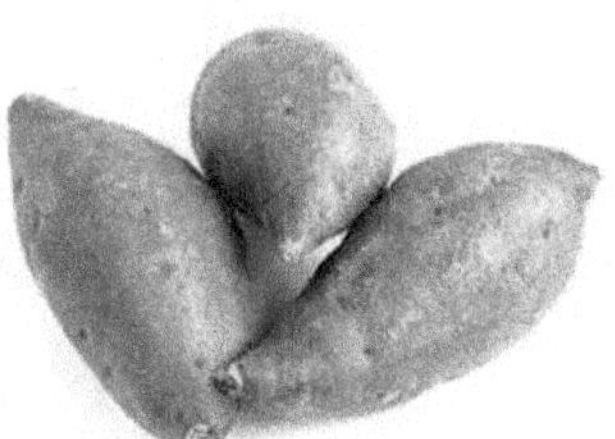

Sweet Potato

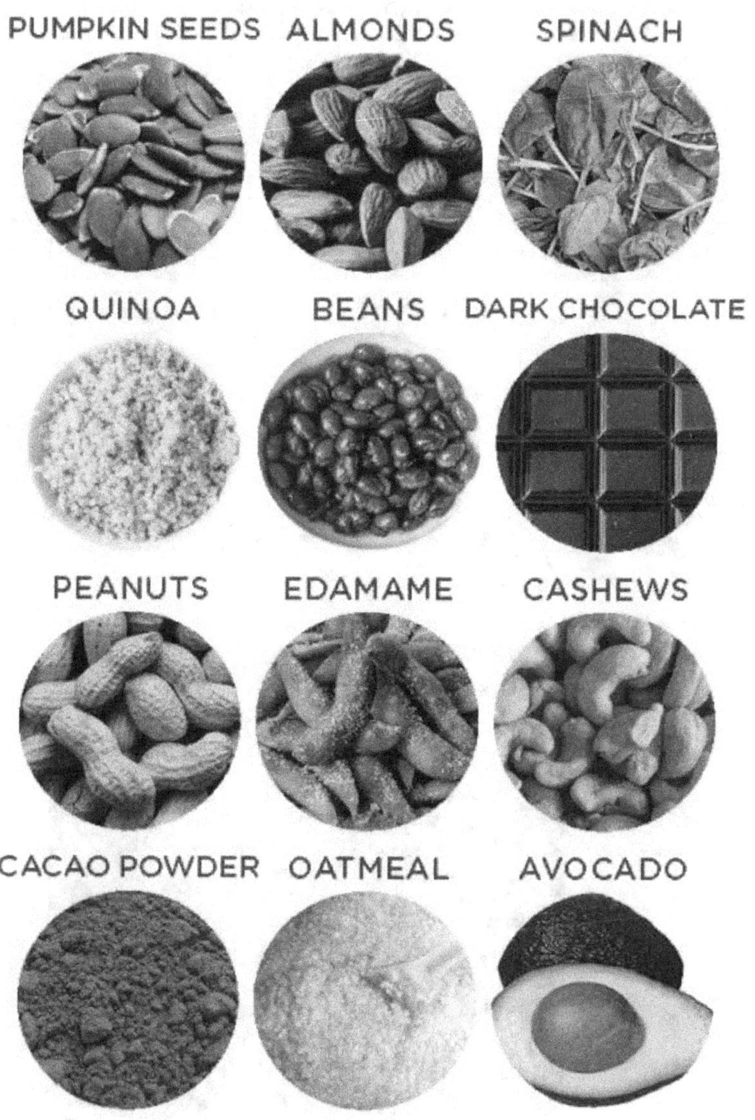

the best food sources
OF MAGNESIUM
PUMPKIN SEEDS
ALMONDS
SPINACH
QUINOA
BEANS
DARK CHOCOLATE
PEANUTS
EDAMAME
CASHEWS
CACAO POWDER
OATMEAL
AVOCADO

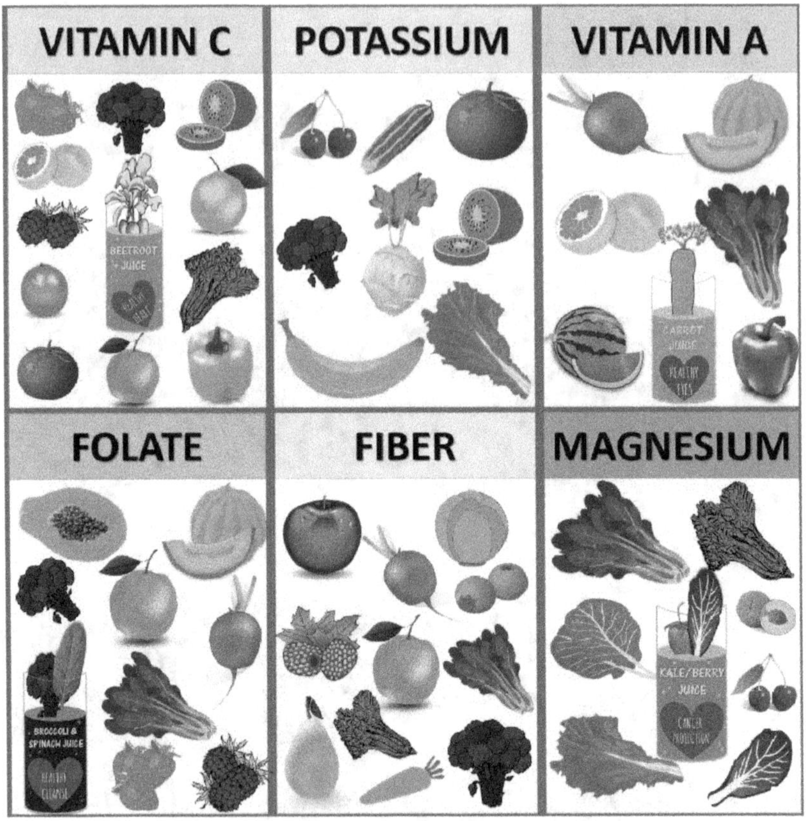
VITAMIN C
POTASSIUM
VITAMIN A
BEETROOT JUICE
CARROT JUICE
FOLATE
FIBER
MAGNESIUM
BROCCOLI & SPINACH JUICE
KALE/BERRY JUICE

No Meat.
No Problem.
Introducing
Chad Byers
Since becoming vegan, he has become stronger and more ripped.
And so can you!
VEGAN
BODYBUILDING
& FITNESS

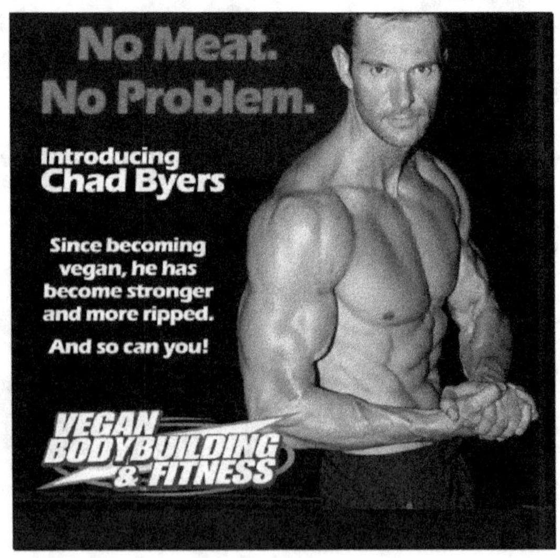

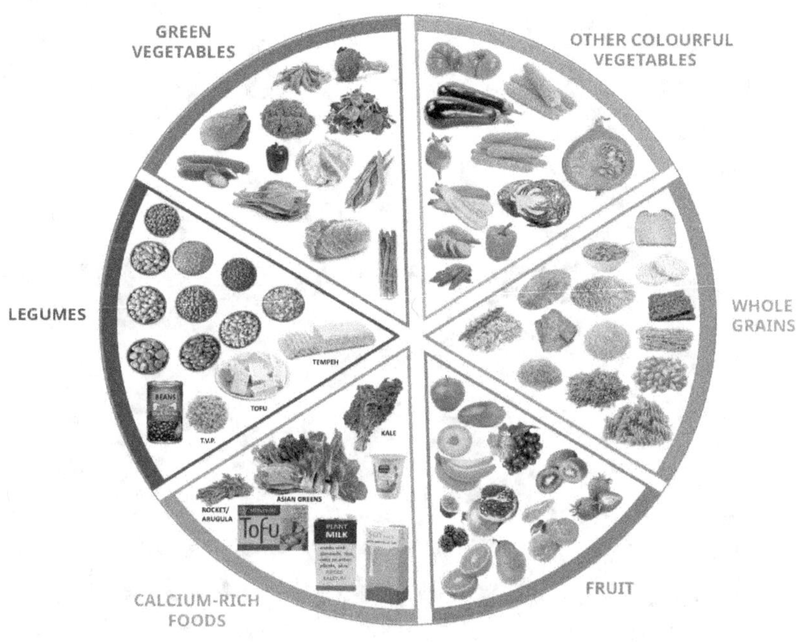

GREEN VEGETABLES
OTHER COLOURFUL VEGETABLES
LEGUMES
WHOLE GRAINS
TEMPEH
KALE
BEANS
T.V.P.
TOFU
ROCKET/ ARUGULA
ASIAN GREENS
Tofu
PLANT MILK
CALCIUM-RICH FOODS
FRUIT

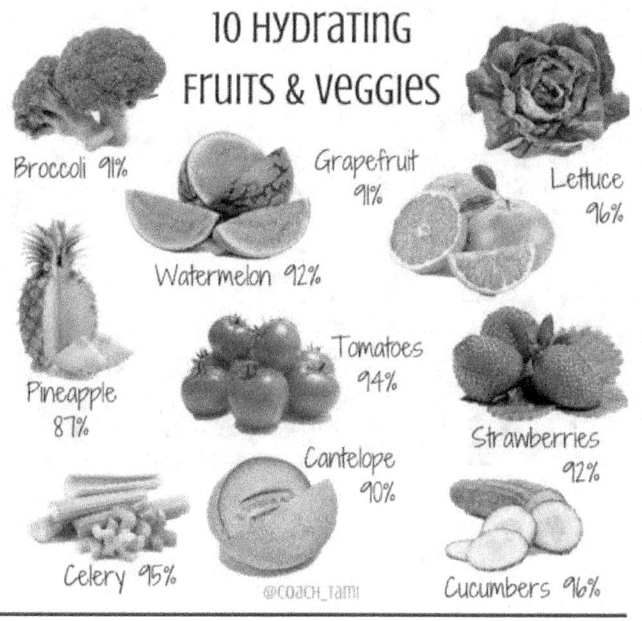

10 HYDRATING FRUITS & VEGGIES
Broccoli 91%
Grapefruit 91%
Lettuce 96%
Watermelon 92%
Pineapple 87%
Tomatoes 94%
Strawberries 92%
Celery 95%
Cantelope 90%
Cucumbers 96%
@coach_tami

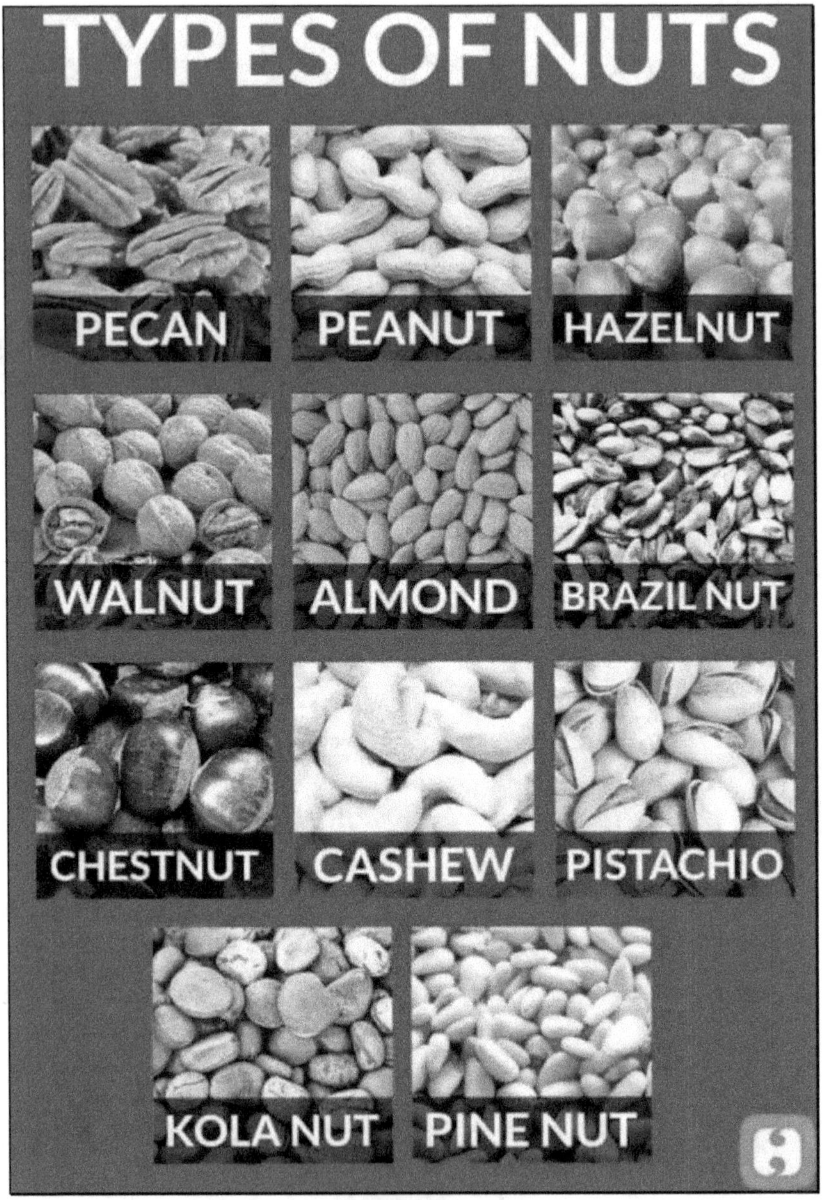
TYPES OF NUTS
PECAN
PEANUT
HAZELNUT
WALNUT
ALMOND
BRAZIL NUT
CHESTNUT
CASHEW
PISTACHIO
KOLA NUT
PINE NUT

vegan

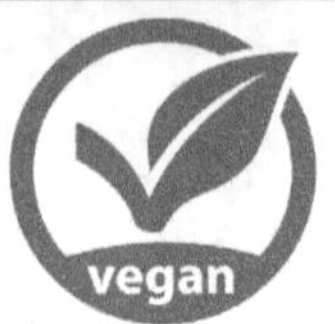

TOP 25
Vegan Protein
SOURCES CHART

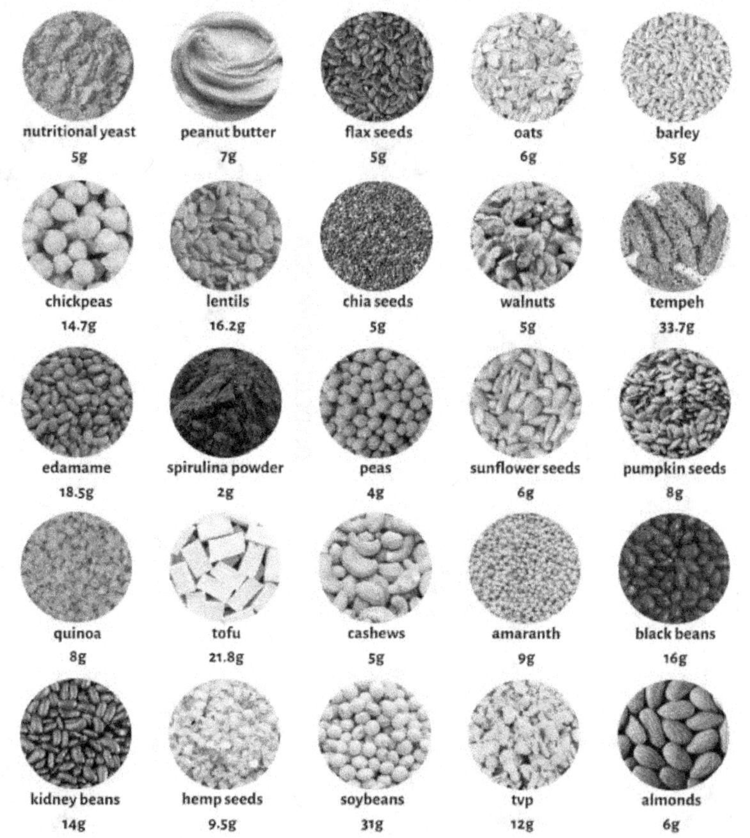

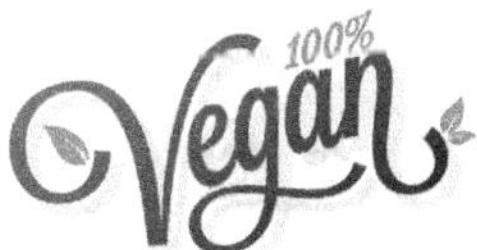

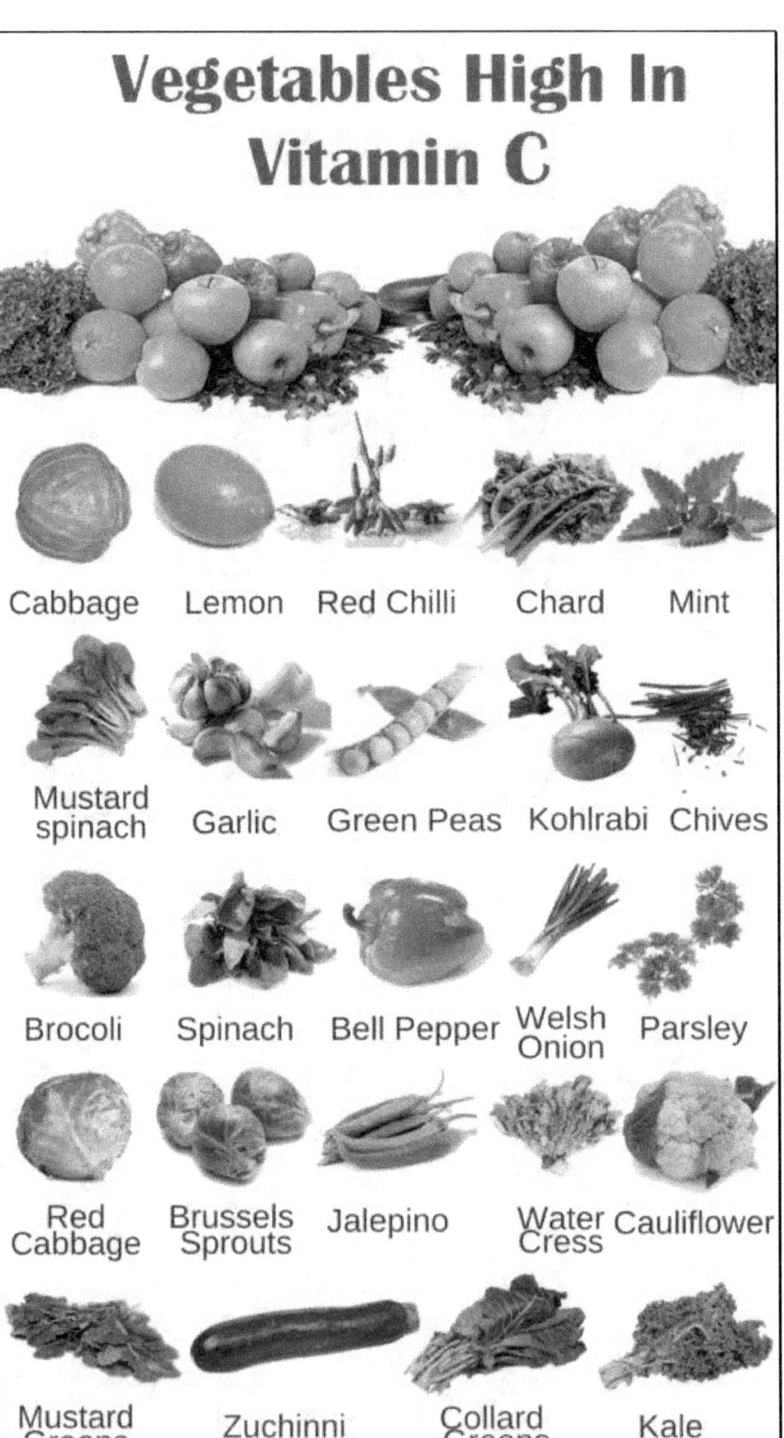

Vegetables High In Vitamin C

Cabbage
Lemon
Red Chilli
Chard
Mint

Mustard spinach
Garlic
Green Peas
Kohlrabi
Chives

Brocoli
Spinach
Bell Pepper
Welsh Onion
Parsley

Red Cabbage
Brussels Sprouts
Jalepino
Water Cress
Cauliflower

Mustard Greens
Zuchinni
Collard Greens
Kale

11 Foods to Improve Brain Function

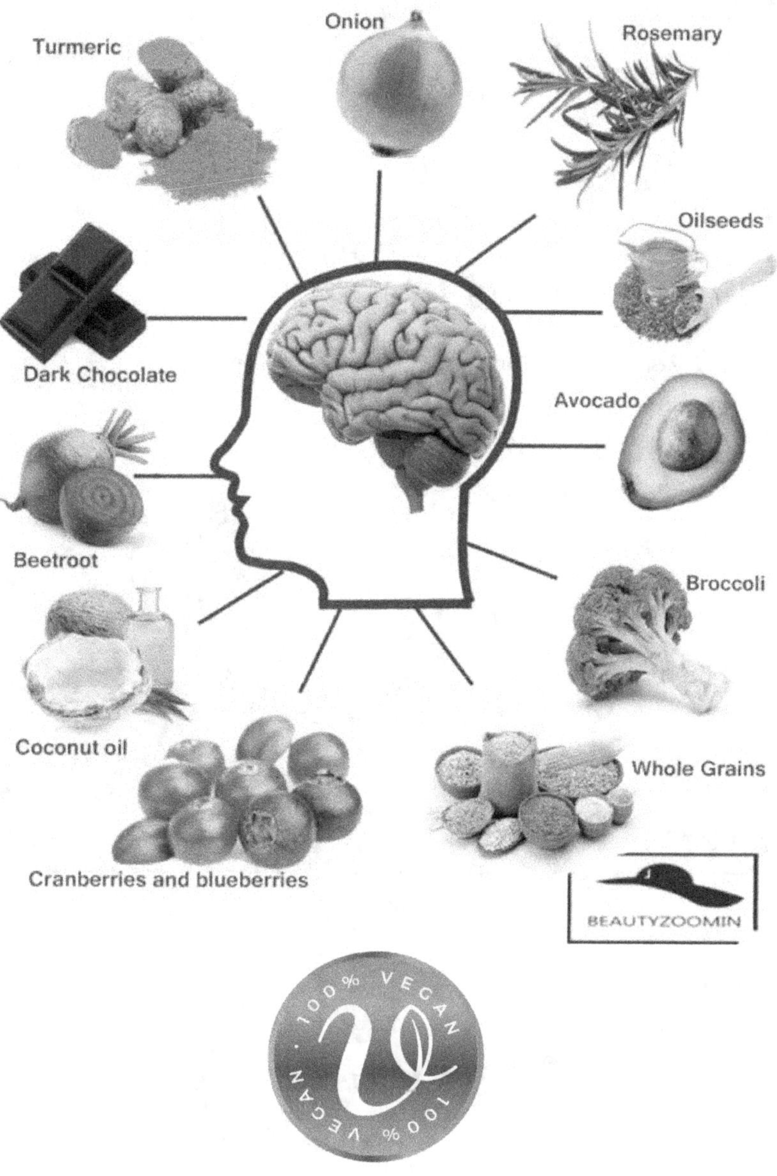

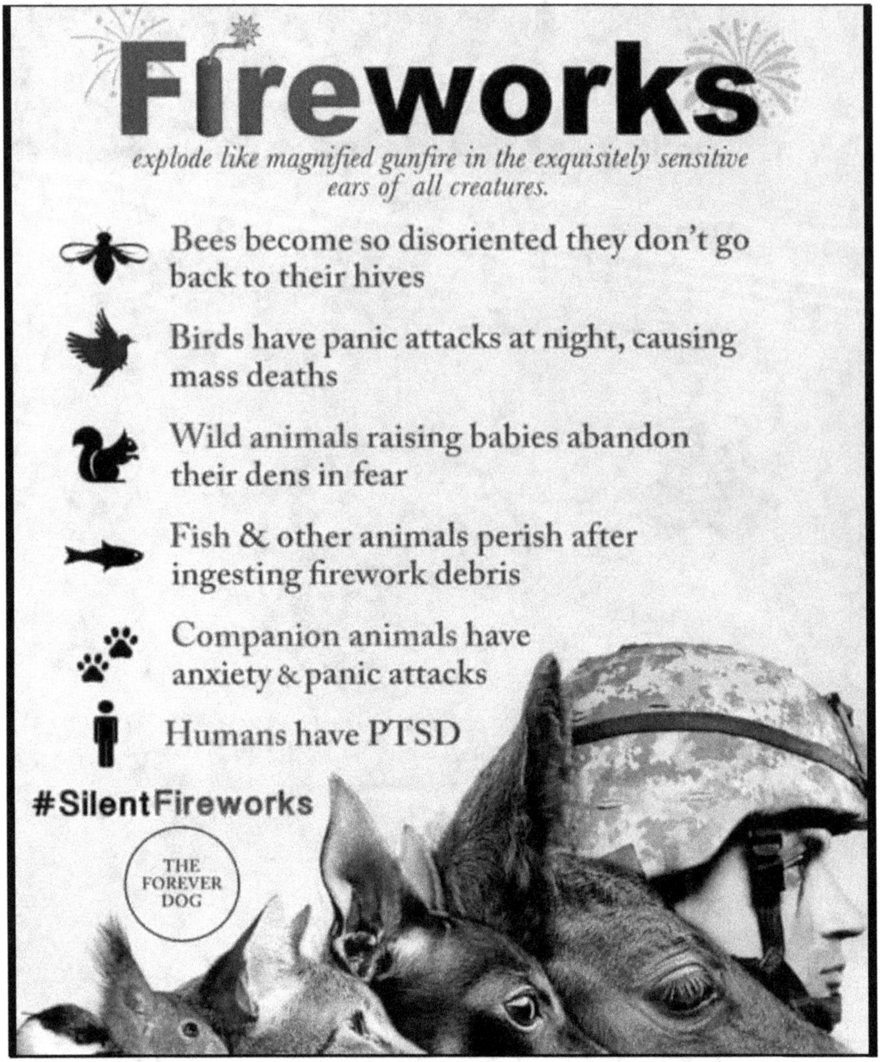

Fireworks
explode like magnified gunfire in the exquisitely sensitive ears of all creatures.

Bees become so disoriented they don't go back to their hives

Birds have panic attacks at night, causing mass deaths

Wild animals raising babies abandon their dens in fear

Fish & other animals perish after ingesting firework debris

Companion animals have anxiety & panic attacks

Humans have PTSD

#SilentFireworks

THE FOREVER DOG

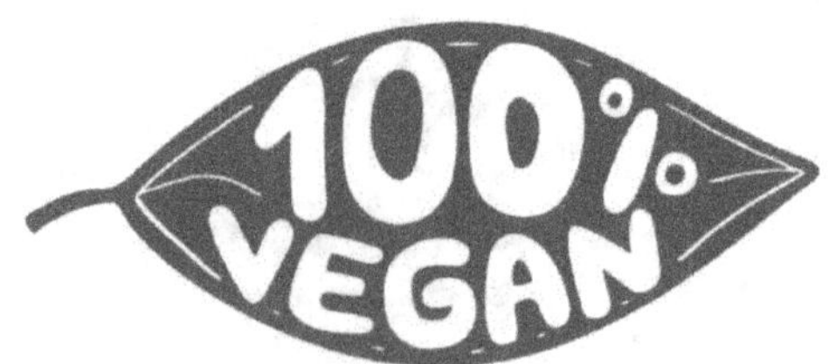

100% VEGAN

About the Author – Tim Mtshali

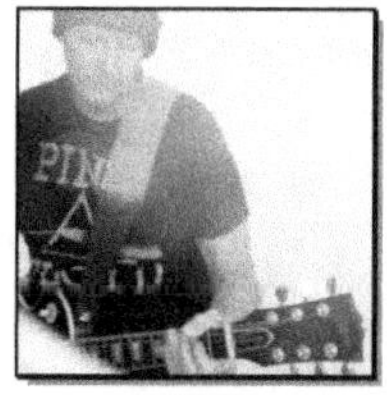

Robin Morris lives in Jeffreys Bay, South Africa. His passion in life is animals. He has written and published a number of books to-date, ranging from fiction to holistic, including animals, humour and surfing. Robin is also an accomplished musician, guitarist, pianist and songwriter with albums available on various online web sites. His genre is primarily rock & blues but he also enjoys acoustic.

Robin's passion for animals began many years ago when he was a Dog Handler in the South African Navy, working with highly intelligent German Shepherds and years later as a Game Guide on a Wildlife Reserve. This obviously led to a lasting relationship with a wide range of animal and birdlife diversity, convincing him of the need to introduce animal education at local school level.

During his twenty something years heading up an Animal Rescue Agency, Robin studied Animal Psychology, specialising in Animal Behaviour Patterns, which provided him with an insight into Animal Dynamics and hence, a lot of material for this book. It is the essence of the written word that captures his passion for writing.   **www.robinmorris.co.za**